T0291699

Healing Psychiatry

Basic Bioethics

Glenn McGee and Arthur Caplan, editors

Healing Psychiatry
Bridging the Science/Humanism Divide

David H. Brendel

The MIT Press
Cambridge, Massachusetts
London, England

First MIT Press paperback edition, 2009

© 2006 Massachusetts Institute of Technology

All rights reserved. No part of this book may be reproduced in any form by any electronic or mechanical means (including photocopying, recording, or information storage and retrieval) without permission in writing from the publisher.

This book was set in Sabon by SPI Publisher Services

Library of Congress Cataloging-in-Publication Data

Brendel, David H.
Healing psychiatry: bridging the science/humanism divide/David H. Brendel.
    p.   m.—(Basic bioethics)
Includes bibliographical references and index.
ISBN 978-0-262-02594-2 (hc. : alk. paper)—978-0-262-51325-8(pb. : alk. paper)
1. Psychiatry—Moral and ethical aspects. 2. Psychiatry—Philosophy.
3. Psychiatric. I. Title. II. Series.
RC455.2.E8B74 2006   174.2'9689—dc22   2005052048

For Becca

In the varied topography of professional practice, there is a high, hard ground where practitioners can make effective use of research-based theory and technique, and there is a swampy lowland where situations are confusing "messes" incapable of technical solution. The difficulty is that the problems of the high ground, however great their technical interest, are often relatively unimportant to clients or to the larger society, while in the swamp are the problems of greatest human concern. Shall the practitioner stay on the high, hard ground where he can practice rigorously, as he understands rigor, but where he is constrained to deal with problems of relatively little social importance? Or shall he descend to the swamp where he can engage the most important and challenging problems if he is willing to forsake technical rigor?

—Donald Schön, *The Reflective Practitioner*

Contents

Series Foreword

We are pleased to present the eighteenth book in the series Basic Bioethics. The series presents innovative works in bioethics to a broad audience and introduces seminal scholarly manuscripts, state-of-the-art reference works, and textbooks. Such broad areas as the philosophy of medicine, advancing genetics and biotechnology, end-of-life care, health and social policy, and the empirical study of biomedical life are engaged.

Glenn McGee
Arthur Caplan

Basic Bioethics Series Editorial Board
Tod S. Chambers
Susan Dorr Goold
Mark Kuczewski
Herman Saatkamp

Foreword

One afternoon, in the drop-in center for homeless women in the derelict part of town where I do my anthropological fieldwork these days, I was sitting at the front table doing a crossword puzzle and chatting with women as they came past. Two women sat at another table side by side. I'd figured out that they were each psychotic. That wasn't too difficult. By the end of the afternoon, one woman was talking out loud to someone who was not present. The other woman picked up her belongings grumpily and walked out. "I've got to get out of here," she said on the way. "I'm diagnosed paranoid schizophrenic. That woman reminds me too much of myself."

The practice of psychiatry is fraught with paradox. Those who are in need of psychiatric help often know one thing clearly, which is that to know that you need help is to know that you cannot trust what you know. To acknowledge that is to acknowledge your doubt about those very things that make you human. And so one cannot pretend that psychiatric diagnosis and interpretation happen in the abstract, that the problem of how to explain and diagnose psychiatric illness is a matter of some neutral, distant science, divorced from the meaning that patients and doctors assign to the words. Is schizophrenia the result of a broken brain or a family drama? The way you answer that question has moral, emotional, and motivational consequences for patients and their families. More perhaps than in any other branch of medicine, the meaning of a psychiatric diagnosis is integrally connected to the outcome of the treatment, because in no other branch of medicine is diagnosis so redolent of implications about the self, and in no other branch of medicine does treatment depend so frankly on the process of self-judgment and self-direction. Yet it is rare to see that relationship recognized in a theoretical model of the underlying principles of the discipline. That is what David Brendel achieves in this book. He rethinks the fundamental principles of psychiatry—what one might imagine as its timeless truths—from the vantage point of their meaning for the individuals that those principles describe.

This is important because there are, in fact, many different models of the cause and nature of mental illness. Schizophrenia is perhaps the most notorious site of the transformation of one model into another. Back when psychoanalysis dominated American psychiatry, back before DSM-III and the biomedical revolution, the dominant American perspective on schizophrenia held that the condition was the result of the patient's own emotional conflict. Such patients were unable to reconcile intense feelings of longing for intimacy with the fear of closeness. Neglect in early childhood and their subsequent intense resentment, fury, and violence drove them into an autistic self-preoccupation from which they yearned for contact but were too terrified to reach out for it. Often, clinicians blamed the mother for delivering conflicting messages of hope and rejection. She was "schizophrenogenic": her own ambivalence paralyzed her child and drove him or her into the clinical impasse of the illness. When psychiatry shifted to a biomedical model of mental illness, the psychodynamic blame associated with the schizophrenogenic mother was seen as an unforgivable sin. Such mothers, psychiatrists realized, had not only had to struggle with losing a child to madness, but with the self-denigration and doubt that came from assuming that they had caused the misery in the first place. And so for many psychiatrists, the new biomedical model had a moral stance. It became not only incorrect, but morally wrong, to see the parents as responsible for their child's illness. In speaking with people diagnosed with schizophrenia and with their parents, then, clinicians—earnestly trying to ward off feelings of blame and guilt on the part of the parents—emphasized the accidental and unexpected, the bad luck that the disorder should strike your family, your son.

Yet this shift to a biomedical model has carried its own moral cost, a cost that I believe, based on my long fieldwork in the psychiatric community, many psychiatrists do not appreciate even now. As schizophrenia became the expression of a broken brain, a mother struggling with losing a child to madness no longer had to blame herself for the tragedy. This hostile, suspicious, terrifying stranger of a son was not her fault. But as she was freed from responsibility, she was also stripped of the capacity to do anything about the train wreck that had been her beloved child. And so, to a large extent, were her child's psychiatrists, whatever they might offer in the way of medication. Schizophrenia became the diagnosis of devastation.

David Brendel argues that psychiatry, as a profession, must learn to think about the process of diagnosis so as to become aware of, and responsive to, the meanings of a diagnosis and the ways patients and their families infer a moral burden. What he does in this book is to sketch out an intellectual scaffolding for this argument, based on philosophical pragmatism. Pragmatism is an appealing philosophical approach because it seems, at least at first, to be simple common sense. First recognize how little you know, it suggests, and do the best you can within your limits. Know what you know, and do not trespass on your ignorance because that is when you falter. First do no harm.

But in fact pragmatism is a very difficult philosophy. It asks you to judge an idea by its consequences, not its principles. To use William James's most famous example, God exists pragmatically because he moves the human heart, not because in some absolute sense he exists independent of our being. Pragmatism asks you not to commit yourself to a single version of the truth, nor even to a single position. It asks you to judge a theory by its consequences, by the way it lives in the minds of those who embrace it.

This is the philosophical approach David Brendel asks us to take toward psychiatric illness. He is persuaded that psychiatric illness is genuinely complex and that many different psychiatric approaches grasp only parts of the underlying reality, pieces of the elephant. But he also believes that different approaches have different consequences for the way patients understand their suffering and the way psychiatrists think about their illness. His goal is to help the profession straddle the ravine between scientific and humanistic perspectives because patients, practitioners, and even scientists are better off if they maintain a rich and complex view of mental illness. Trained as a philosopher, he builds a philosophical foundation for this straddling from Charles Sanders Peirce, William James, and John

Dewey. These men believed deeply in the process of the scientific enterprise, but they also believed that any plausible science had to acknowledge the messy complexity of the human context. Brendel draws from them four main points: an insistence on the practical dimension of all scientific inquiry; the pluralistic nature of the phenomena studied by science; the need to involve many participants, many perspectives; and the provisional and flexible character of scientific explanation.

What that means for the practice of psychiatry, he argues, is radical: that psychiatric explanations are valid only insofar as they promote beneficial real-world results. He argues that in some fundamental sense, the truth of a theory must be understood as a relationship between what the psychiatrist says and what happens to the patient. The truth of an explanation then depends in part on the way the patient hears it and responds. Because of this, he argues, it is not only ethically but scientifically wrong to limit the field to one side of the debate between scientific and humanistic approaches to mental illness, and it is wrong to presume that theories are complete or adequate. The patient must participate as an agent in the treatment process, as someone who will interpret the diagnosis and act on his or her interpretation, and whose response to some theory serves as a judgment on the theory's value. Such an approach maintains a complex model of mental illness that demands an array of conceptual tools and intellectual orientations, an approach that does not reject neuroscience but that adopts it as one level of many in interpreting and engaging human distress.

Let me return to the puzzle of the street. The drop-in center makes the clinical importance of negotiating the meaning of diagnosis brutally clear. As a client, one rapidly learns that being crazy is the worst possible identity that you can assume. Flagrantly psychotic women disturb other women's conversations, disrupt the staff, and cannot be trusted by other clients because their behavior cannot be predicted. No one likes them. I was chatting to a woman one afternoon about her friendships, and asked whether she was friends with a women sitting nearby, who would occasionally declaim to the wall. She was pretty obviously schizophrenic. The woman I was speaking with was no stranger to psychiatry. She's been hospitalized several times for suicide attempts and cutting, she spoke with pleasure about her therapist, and she'd comfortably explained that she was diagnosed with depression and borderline personality, neither of which count on the street as "crazy." "*Her?*" she asked disdainfully. "She doesn't need any friends. She talks plenty to herself."

For those on the street, "crazy" means being an obviously psychotic person you don't want to talk with, who creates trouble for you, and to whom people are mean, aggressive, and violent. Here "crazy" becomes a stand-in for the worst thing that the street can do to you, which is to render you unfit for human contact. This is the literal interpretation of madness as a "broken brain."

And so many women refuse to accept any suggestion that they need the psychiatrist's help. "I am a person," announced another woman I often saw talking to the air, "who would *never* allow myself to go crazy." In fact, you can get housing easily on the street if you have a serious psychotic disorder. It is far from easy to get housed without a so-called disability. "You can get housing if you're crazy, addicted, or you got a job," one woman remarked, ticking off the options. "I ain't got a job and I'm not crazy, so I'm working on addicted." Many women not only do not accept such housing, but will even refuse to "pretend" to be psychiatrically ill so as to be eligible for that housing. That illness renders you eligible is well known. But many women who are obviously psychotic say that they wouldn't lie about being "crazy" just to get that housing. "I'm not *that* kind of a person," said a woman who had just finished explaining to me how hard life is in the shelters because she believes that she is constantly pursued by a large, threatening mob.

The way these women understand a diagnosis is central to the way they choose to negotiate their relationship with psychiatric services. If they could learn to hold a more complex model of mental illness, as something that may wax and wane, as something that might be influenced by social context, and as something that could change with care—we might be able to get them the care that they now reject. They might not read Brendel's book. But if the message he imparts would filter down to the social world in which they are embedded, they might find more hope than they are able to at present.

T. M. Luhrmann
Chicago

Acknowledgments

This book is the culmination of many years of interdisciplinary study in psychiatry, philosophy, and ethics. I first developed a youthful fascination with this area as a student of Maurice Natanson at Yale College, where I had many formative learning experiences in the seminars on psychiatry and existentialism that he offered in the years before his death. As a student at Harvard Medical School, I had the good fortune to take Ed Hundert's seminar on parallel forms of reasoning in philosophy, psychiatry, and neuroscience. His book *Philosophy, Psychiatry, and Neuroscience: Three Approaches to the Mind* inspired me to pursue further interdisciplinary work and to take a leave of absence from medical school to pursue graduate study in philosophy at the University of Chicago. My work at Chicago was funded by the Pew Charitable Trusts. The members of my dissertation committee (Arnold Davidson, Michael Forster, Fred Ovsiew, and Bill Wimsatt), the leaders of the university's Program in Medicine, Arts, and the Social Sciences (Godfrey Getz, Roberta Siegel, and Stanley Yachnin), and the dean of students at the Pritzker School of Medicine (Norma Waggoner) were instrumental in helping me to build a career in philosophy and psychiatry.

After completing psychiatry residency training at Massachusetts General Hospital and McLean Hospital, I spent a year as a Faculty Fellow in the Harvard University Center for Ethics and the Professions, where I received funding from the Eugene P. Beard scholarship fund to continue my work on philosophy, ethics, and psychiatry. During that year, I was fortunate to work with ethicists like Nomy Arpaly and Bob Truog, who helped me to hone my thinking and move my work toward an in-depth exploration of professionalism and ethics in psychiatric practice. I extend special thanks to Dennis Thompson for his remark-able leadership of the center and wholehearted support of my work. In the year following my fellowship in the Harvard ethics center, I had the good fortune to receive ongoing funding for my work from the American Psychiatric Association/Wyeth-Ayerst M.D./Ph.D. Psychiatric Research Fellowship.

My professional and academic homes for the last several years have been at Harvard Medical School, McLean Hospital, Massachusetts General Hospital, and the Boston Psychoanalytic Institute. The remark-able talent of the individuals in these institutions and the compassionate nature of the clinical care they provide—not to mention the extraor-dinary wealth of academic and intellectual resources these institutions make available—have profoundly shaped my thinking about what psy-chiatry is and what it ought to be in the future. In a short space, it would be impossible to express my deep thanks to all my mentors and col-leagues in these institutions who have helped me to shape the ideas that I develop in this book. I especially thank the following individuals for their support of this work: Ross Baldessarini, Alec Bodkin, Bruce Cohen, Shelly Greenfield, Les Havens, Kathy Sanders, Ted Stern, and Alex Vuckovic. I am grateful to Les Havens and Ted Stern for their careful readings of early versions of the manuscript and helpful suggestions about how to revise it. Many thanks as well to my colleagues in the Association for the Advancement of Philosophy and Psychiatry, particu-larly Nassir Ghaemi, Jennifer Radden, John Sadler, and Peter Zachar.

I appreciate the permission to reprint portions of several of my pre-viously published articles, which have appeared in the *Harvard Review of Psychiatry*, *Journal of Clinical Ethics*, *Journal of Medicine and Philosophy*, and *Philosophy, Psychiatry, & Psychology*:

Portions of chapters 1, 2, 3, and 8 previously appeared in D. H. Brendel, "Healing Psychiatry: A Pragmatic Approach to Bridging the Science/Humanism Divide," *Harvard Review of Psychiatry* 12 (2004):150–157. Reproduced by permission of Taylor and Francis, Inc., http://www.taylorandfrancis.com.

Portions of chapters 1, 2, and 3 previously appeared in D. H. Brendel, "Reductionism, Eclecticism, and Pragmatism in Psychiatry: The Dialectic of Clinical Explanation," *Journal of Medicine and Philosophy* 28 (2003):563–580. Reproduced by permission of Taylor and Francis, Inc., http://www.taylorandfrancis.com.

Portions of chapters 1, 2, and 8 previously appeared in D. H. Brendel, "The Ethics of Diagnostic and Therapeutic Paradigm Choice in Psychiatry," *Harvard Review of Psychiatry* 10 (2002):47–50. Reproduced by permission of Taylor and Francis, Inc., http://www.taylorandfrancis.com.

Portions of chapter 3 previously appeared in D. H. Brendel et al., " 'In Sleep I Almost Never Grope': Blindness, Neuropsychiatric Deficits, and a Chaotic Upbringing," *Harvard Review of Psychiatry* 9 (2001): 178–188. Reproduced by permission of Taylor and Francis, Inc., http://www.taylorandfrancis.com.

Portions of chapter 3 previously appeared in D. H. Brendel et al., " 'I See Dead People': Overcoming Psychic Numbness," *Harvard Review of Psychiatry* 10 (2002):166–178. Reproduced by permission of Taylor and Francis, Inc., http://www.taylorandfrancis.com.

Portions of chapter 3 previously appeared in D. H. Brendel, "Complications to Consent," *Journal of Clinical Ethics* 14 (2003): 90–94. © The Journal of Clinical Ethics, 2003. All Rights Reserved.

Portions of chapter 4 previously appeared in D. H. Brendel, "Philosophy of Mind in the Clinic: The Relation between Causal and Meaningful Explanation in Psychiatry," *Harvard Review of Psychiatry* 8 (2000):184–191. Reproduced by permission of Taylor and Francis, Inc., http://www.taylorandfrancis.com.

Portions of chapter 7 previously appeared in D. H. Brendel, "Multifactorial Causation of Mental Disorders: A Proposal to Improve the DSM," *Harvard Review of Psychiatry* 9 (2001):42–45. Reproduced by permission of Taylor and Francis, Inc., http://www.taylorandfrancis.com.

Portions of chapter 7 previously appeared in D. H. Brendel, "A Pragmatic Consideration of the Relation between Depression and Melancholia," *Philosophy, Psychiatry, & Psychology* 10 (2003):53–55. Reproduced by permission of Johns Hopkins University Press.

I am deeply grateful to my editor at The MIT Press, Clay Morgan, and to the editors of the Basic Bioethics series, Glenn McGee and Arthur

Caplan, for providing a home for this book and for creating a space where novel approaches to contemporary bioethics are welcomed and developed. I thank Tanya Luhrmann for helping to clarify what is "disordered" in contemporary American psychiatry and for writing the foreword to this book.

On a personal note, I thank George Fishman for all of his wonderful guidance and wisdom over the years and for his helpful critique of a version of the manuscript of this book. Finally, I thank my entire family for their love and all they have done to make this book possible. I am especially grateful to my parents, Robert and Jane, my brothers, Gary and Michael, and my wife's family, Joel, Cess, and Stephanie Weintraub. My son, Isaac, was born as I worked on the book in 2004, and he inspired me not only to make it better but also to get it done in a timely way so I would have extra time with him on weekends. My wife, Becca, has believed in me and in this project from its earliest inception, and her constructive readings of many versions of this book were invaluable. She is everything to me, and it is to her that the book is dedicated.

Introduction

The human sciences at the beginning of the twenty-first century remain mired in a quiet but serious and abiding conceptual crisis. Nowhere is this crisis more urgent than the area in which I practice, psychiatry, which faces an ongoing ethical challenge to define what it means to be a human subject in an increasingly scientific era of genetics, neurobiology, and psychopharmacology—and in a fast-paced world that craves self-help books and that seeks the kind of quick fix that popular television psychologists dispense to millions of their viewers each day. Thoughtful, deliberative, tentative accounts of human experience and suffering are hard to come by these days. Our society has grown more impatient to find the gene or the drug or the manual or the website that will explain and help to resolve our most profound existential anxieties. In the rush to understand, explain, and treat with new rapid-fire technologies, many psychiatrists have disengaged from more plodding, uncertain, and ambiguous forms of approaching patients, such as insight-oriented psychotherapy and psychoanalysis. Empirical science has led to some astonishing discoveries and cutting-edge psychiatric treatments that were unimaginable to previous generations. But what, we may ask, have we sacrificed along the way? What role might individual subjectivity and humanism still play in contemporary medical and psychiatric science? How might clinical practitioners of these disciplines apply the emerging scientific technologies judiciously while respecting the dignity and individualized needs of each of their patients?

These questions have bothered and fascinated me for many years. They first struck me in a deeply personal way at the very same time that they captured my intellectual curiosity in medical school and graduate school in philosophy. At that time, I was in my midtwenties and in a state of emotional chaos following a painful breakup with a girlfriend. The breakup, my obsessive focus on academic work, and my exciting but precarious plan to take a leave of absence from my medical school studies to pursue graduate work in philosophy left me in a state of confusion, inner turmoil, self-doubt, and sleeplessness. Feeling that I had no place else to turn, I made an appointment with a psychiatrist at the university health service and began an arduous process that would lead to years of psychotherapy and four-times-per-week psychoanalysis. It solidified my long-standing aspirations to pursue a career at the interface of philosophy, ethics, and clinical psychiatry, and it deepened my fascination with a broad spectrum of abstract and practical questions about the human mind and its pathologies. Would future discoveries in genetics and neuroscience eventually explain why I had become so overwhelmed and obsessive? Would the right medication targeting relevant neurotransmitters prevent me from having to live through future episodes of anxiety and despair? Did the content of my dreams and my free associations in therapy sessions tell me anything meaningful about my emotional state and about my disquieting pattern of reacting to a difficult break up?

As I pondered my situation, I wondered to what extent my struggles were the result of a biological vulnerability to an anxiety disorder. Was psychotropic medication necessary to correct an inborn derangement of brain neurotransmitter functioning? What was the role of complicated family dynamics, including my nervousness and guilt that grew out of a daunting set of parental expectations for my success as well as the vigorous competition I had experienced from siblings who challenged my pride of place in the family? Was it my inborn temperament or my early childhood experiences (or both, or neither) that had rendered me susceptible as a young adult to feeling distraught when an intimate relationship went bad? Perhaps psychotherapy and psychoanalysis were the principal agents of personal growth as I matured into my thirties, married, launched a career, and started a family. On the other hand, is it conceivable that there was no bedrock explanation for the complicated ups and downs, the unforeseen twists and turns, which my life had taken? In essence, is there, or is there not, a plausible and coherent account of these developments? And if there is a coherent account, how does that account need to be revised as I confront new psychological challenges that have emerged in my thirties? These questions reverberated with those I asked myself about my own patients during my years in medical school and psychiatric residency, and which I continue to ask myself every day in the course of clinical practice.

This depiction of my personal struggles raises universal questions: what (if any) concepts might account for why people suffer as they do and would allow psychiatrists to diagnose and treat them in a beneficial and humane fashion? In the era of genetics, neuroimaging, and psychophar-macology, will the concepts of the biological and behavioral sciences be adequate to this task? Or are people so complex that the concepts of the humanities and the liberal arts will remain at the core of clinical psychia-try regardless of how far psychiatric neuroscience happens to advance in the future? Is psychiatry an empirical science that aims to diagnose and treat abnormal human behavior, or is it a form of humanism that addresses the inner workings and meanings of people's subjective experi-ences and existential concerns? Motivated equally by my existential anx-iety and intellectual curiosity as a student, I began to immerse myself in these academic and practical questions—and quickly discovered that there are longstanding and deep divisions between the science and the humanism of psychiatry. Over the years since then, as I built my career in psychiatry and worked to heal some of the emotional wounds in my own life, I remained intrigued and troubled by the failure of psychiatry to heal itself. The field continues to be torn apart by strong and divergent pulls toward a science that studies brain functioning and a humanism that studies the mind in its broad social and cultural context.

But these conceptual ruptures and rifts in psychiatry provide some unique opportunities for synthesis and integration. The process of seek-ing the conceptual reparation of psychiatry is now the core ethical mis-sion of a field that is trying to heal itself so that it is better equipped to heal the patients whom it aims to serve. Healing psychiatry is about resolving the conceptual dichotomy between science and humanism so that patients in the twenty-first century can receive the best possible men-tal health care. The title of this book is meant to capture both of these aspects of the healing process. My principal aim in the book is to heal certain dimensions of the science/humanism rupture by delineating a novel approach to psychiatric reasoning.

The healing of psychiatry demands a thorough appreciation of the field's explanatory models, which are the sets of fundamental concepts and systematic approaches to understanding and treating mental illnesses that psychiatrists use to ground their clinical practice. Explanatory models in psychiatry reflect what clinicians deem valuable in rendering a person's behavior intelligible and thus help to guide treatment choices for mental disorders. Most current explanatory models in psychiatry are either primarily scientific or primarily humanistic. The former are attractive inasmuch as they aim to justify clinical explanations and treatments by way of empirical evidence and scientific rigor, but they are flawed inasmuch as they tend to restrict options for diagnostic and therapeutic paradigm choice. The latter have the advantage of acknowledging the complex, subjective, and multifaceted features of most mental disorders, but they are imperfect because they often lack a coherent and well-defined basis in empirically derived scientific evidence.

The scientific and humanistic approaches stand in a dialectical relationship to one another insofar as psychiatric clinicians often find themselves moving from one approach to its antithesis, ultimately striving to forge a synthesis that satisfies the clinical needs of the moment. Dialectical reasoning, which can be traced to the early nineteenth-century work of German philosopher G. W. F. Hegel, entails serious consideration of both sides of a conceptual dilemma, recognition of the possible relevance of both sides, and active efforts to articulate the appropriate relation between them. The dialectic is an interactive, dynamic process in which each side of the conceptual divide constantly informs, shapes, and responds to the opposing side. Dialectical reasoning is well suited to the challenges of psychiatry, in which the conceptual foundations of practice remain in dispute, the causes of symptoms are frequently indeterminable, diagnosis depends largely on patients' self-reports of symptoms, and appropriate treatment of most clinical syndromes remains a matter of trial and error. In the absence of a broad consensus regarding appropriate concepts and methodologies to be employed in their work, clinical psychiatrists need to tolerate ambiguity and uncertainty as they try to integrate diverse scientific and humanistic concepts in a dialectical and ethical manner.

This is the most basic challenge that psychiatrists of all stripes face on the contemporary scene. How are they to proceed when they greet and embark on a course of treatment with a complex individual who presents his or her current struggles and dilemmas, past experiences and relationships, and longstanding patterns of coping with conflict, stress, and loss? This question becomes all the more daunting and complicated when considerations of biology—perhaps in the form of response to prescribed medications, substance abuse, neuropsychiatric illness, abnormalities on brain scans, or family history of mental disorders—are factored into the equation. The psychiatrist must organize an enormous mass of clinical data, form plausible hypotheses about the origins of the patient's distress, and develop treatment recommendations to help relieve the patient's suffering. This multifaceted process requires paying careful attention to an incredibly broad array of biological, psychological, and interpersonal considerations. At the same time, the clinical psychiatrist always must remain aware of his or her limitations and mindful of the fact that the patient is in some sense entirely unfathomable.

The main argument I will develop in this book is that pragmatic values can help to transcend the science/humanism divide in modern-day psychiatry. What does this claim amount to? The work of classical American pragmatists (including such thinkers as Charles Sanders Peirce, William James, and John Dewey) and the work of contemporary pragmatic bioethicists have suggested that certain core ideas and principles ought to guide the pursuit of science in general, and medical sciences in particular. These thinkers urge us to pay close attention to the practical applications of scientific study, the multiplicity of phenomena that render such study useful, the participation of many individuals in formulating collaborative and workable hypotheses, and the provisional nature of scientific understanding. Along these lines, pragmatism in modern-day psychiatry can be understood as a clinical sensibility and methodology that aims for favorable treatment outcomes for patients by respecting the practical, pluralistic, participatory, and provisional aspects of psychiatric explanation. Clinical pragmatism demands that psychiatrists have the skill and flexibility to employ multiple explanatory concepts (spanning the entire biopsychosocial spectrum) in an interactive and collaborative process with patients, which under most circumstances can lead to open-ended but useful clinical explanations and treatment plans. It is by way of clinical pragmatism that the conceptual wounds in psychiatry and the emotional wounds in the lives of individuals can begin to heal.

This book explores these themes from clinical and theoretical standpoints. Chapter 1 delineates the dialectic of science and humanism in contemporary philosophy of science and clinical psychiatry. Chapter 2 presents an argument for working through and transcending this dialectic by applying basic principles of classical American pragmatism and contemporary pragmatic bioethics to psychiatric reasoning and practice. Chapter 3 contains several psychiatric case histories that highlight the benefits of integrating science and humanism in an ethical, patient-centered, and pragmatic fashion. These first three chapters lay out the basic argument that a deeply problematic science/humanism dichotomy continues to plague clinical psychiatry, that this dichotomy can best be managed and overcome by employing principles of clinical pragmatism, and that clinical case histories provide a clear rationale and justification for applying the principles of pragmatism to everyday psychiatric practice.

The remainder of the book unfolds as follows. Chapter 4 includes a discussion of the relevance of pragmatism to current philosophy of mind and the mind/brain relation in psychiatry. Chapter 5 traces the evolution of Sigmund Freud's understanding of the mind/brain relation and his pragmatic move from clinical neurology to psychology, a shift that retains significant contemporary relevance. Chapter 6 is a plea, based on pragmatic values, for an ongoing separation of neurology and psychiatry as distinct and autonomous clinical disciplines. Chapter 7 contains an argument for a liberal and flexible, yet scientifically informed, notion of causal explanation in clinical psychiatry and presents implications of these pragmatic values for psychiatric diagnosis in general, and for the American Psychiatric Association's *Diagnostic and Statistical Manual of Mental Disorders* (DSM) in particular. The future of psychiatry is explored in chapter eight, where the principles of clinical pragmatism are applied to a wide range of ethical concerns and challenges in psychiatric training and research. This final chapter contains reflections on the origins and the vicissitudes of our stubborn tendency to divide persons into objects for scientific study and subjects of irreducibly human experience, and it explores the promise and limits of clinical pragmatism today and in the years to come.

1

Science and Humanism in Psychiatry

Clashing conceptual approaches have left the science of psychiatry deeply wounded at the start of the new millennium. Competing urges to think of human mental suffering as comprehensible and amenable to scientific formulation, or as hopelessly complex and beyond the reach of scientific analysis, have torn at the fabric of the field for many years. Tanya Luhrmann's anthropological study of American psychiatry in the 1990s, conducted in hospitals and clinics around the country, revealed a field very much in search of itself and increasingly divided along scientific and humanistic lines. Her long-term study resulted in 2000 in the publication of her influential book *Of Two Minds: The Growing Disorder in American Psychiatry*, in which she evocatively described her observations over several years of the inpatient and outpatient psychiatric care that patients received in private and public hospitals throughout the United States.

In the course of her study, Luhrmann found a pervasive and worsening split between biomedical and psychodynamic psychiatry, with the former rapidly replacing the latter due to a variety of considerations, not the least of which were financial constraints on psychotherapy that were imposed by insurance companies and managed-care organizations in the 1990s. Biomedical psychiatry research demonstrated that new psychotropic medications had become safer and more effective than their predecessors, and use of these agents empowered psychiatrists to decrease the length of patients' stays on inpatient psychiatric units from many months to a week or two. In the process, long-term psychotherapy on inpatient units had been rendered obsolete—and by the 1990s most insurance companies stopped paying for it anyway. Psychiatric residents, whose training mostly takes place in the hospital setting, were taught to simplify their clinical formulations by focusing on diagnosis of observable symptoms rather than on descriptions of the complexities of a patient's past and current life experiences and interpersonal relationships. If a patient could be diagnosed with major depression on the basis of a constellation of symptoms (e.g., sad mood, apathy, insomnia, and suicidal ideation), and if the symptoms could be reversed quickly with an antidepressant medication, then in-depth psychotherapy would be unnecessary and the patient could be discharged from the hospital quickly and at a relatively low cost.

While many psychiatrists in training were comfortably adopting their new role as diagnosticians and psychopharmacologists, Luhrmann noted, others were profoundly disturbed by the trend toward simplifying clinical formulations and reducing patients' personal struggles to a list of biologically treatable symptoms. These psychiatrists felt alienated from reductive trends in biomedically oriented psychiatric training and practice, and they largely gravitated toward working in the outpatient clinics, where it was more feasible to get to know patients over a long period of time and to conduct psychodynamic psychotherapy. But even in outpatient settings, the forces of managed care were intensifying and placing limitations on the nature and length of treatment. Psychodynamic psychiatrists preserved a robust sense of the fundamental complexity of the human mind and unconscious motivation, but they were becoming isolated from the mainstream trends toward biomedical diagnosis and treatment.

In addition, Luhrmann pointed out that, like biomedical psychiatrists, psychodynamic psychiatrists looked at impossibly complex human phenomena and attempted to organize, simplify, and reduce them so that they could treat their patients. Their concepts, of course, differed significantly: biomedical psychiatrists attended to somatic symptoms and medication treatments, while psychodynamic clinicians focused on such concepts as traumatic memory, unconscious fantasy, and transference of emotional reactions from the past to situations in the present. Both strove to impose order and coherence on the mess of human existence by developing a set of concepts and therapeutic tools that could be applied in the clinic. In that way, practitioners at both ends of the biomedical/psychodynamic spectrum had developed a common but potentially problematic response to the mystery of human life and psychiatric illness. "The real story of twentieth-century psychiatry," Luhrmann (2000, 212) wrote, "is how complex mental illness is, how difficult it is to treat, and how, in the face of this complexity, people cling to coherent explanations like poor swimmers to a raft." By imposing order on chaos in this way, the biomedical psychiatrist and psychodynamic psychotherapist developed much-needed treatments, but also ran the risk of excluding important human phenomena from their clinical formulations.

Here Luhrmann pointed to the critical dimension of the current disorder in American psychiatry. The major conceptual divide that now confronts psychiatry is between a respect for human complexity (which we can attempt to describe but cannot fully systematize) and the commitments of the behavioral sciences (which aim to categorize, explain, and predict human behavior empirically). Luhrmann argued that clinical psychiatrists may choose to affiliate with the biomedical or the psychodynamic camp in the field, but she also suggested that each practitioner—regardless of his or her theoretical orientation—inevitably becomes entangled in the science/humanism debate. To practice effectively, psychiatrists must acknowledge the dual impulses toward seeing patients as basically intelligible, whether from the biomedical or psychodynamic standpoint, and toward viewing them as irreducibly complex subjects who are fundamentally beyond the reach of rigorous scientific explanation or prediction. Contemporary clinical psychiatrists cannot choose between science and humanism in the way that they can choose between using medications or psychotherapy. Instead, they necessarily face the challenge of tolerating and working intimately with the ambiguities and paradoxes of patients' clinical presentations, in all their scientific and humanistic richness.

Questions about how psychiatric clinicians can meet this challenge resonate with some of the central questions in contemporary philosophy of science. Is the natural world understandable in terms of a set of unified scientific principles and theories? Or is it so complex and pluralistic as to defy scientific analysis? One of the most vigorous and contentious debates in the contemporary philosophy of science crystallizes around these questions. Proponents of the essential unity of knowledge, such as biologist Edward O. Wilson (1998), suggest that facts and theories can be linked in order to create a "common groundwork of explanation" spanning all the natural sciences (including biology, chemistry, and physics) and ultimately subsuming the social sciences and humanities as well; Wilson refers to this idea as "consilience." Opponents of this approach believe that the complexity of the world does not lend itself to such simplification or reduction. Philosopher Frederick Olafson (2001) criticized Wilson's approach for its dogmatic faith in the unifying power of natural science and called this attitude "scientism." Philosopher John Dupré (1993) argued for the essential disunity of knowledge on the basis of our limited cognitive and technological capacities, and on the basis of the profound complexity of the natural world; this he called the fundamental "disorder of things."

This theoretical debate has major implications for clinical explanation and treatment methodology in medicine and psychiatry. Clinicians must acknowledge the complexity of human illness but also strive for scientific coherence in clinical practice. The impulse toward science in psychiatry leads researchers to investigate the root causes of mental disorders by employing emerging technologies ranging from genetics to neuroimaging to psychopharmacology. This same impulse leads psychiatric clinicians to attempt to diagnose and treat their patients by organizing diverse clinical data, postulating that certain groupings of symptoms constitute a well-defined syndrome, establishing a diagnosis, and treating with empirically validated therapies. For example, a set of symptoms such as elevated mood, inflated self-esteem, agitation, and decreased need for sleep constitutes the syndrome of mania, which in the current parlance establishes the diagnosis of bipolar disorder and suggests that appropriate treatment would include mood-stabilizing medication.

When working as scientists, psychiatric researchers and clinicians both aim to establish a unified view of psychiatric illness that links the laboratory to the clinic. A unified view of bipolar disorder would include coherent connections among genetic predispositions, structural and biochemical dysfunction in relevant brain regions, symptoms that result directly from these abnormalities, and clinical interventions that might reverse or ameliorate the disturbance. The social or psychological aspects

of the condition could be best understood in terms of their manifestations in the brain—for instance, the grandiosity and impulsive behavior
of patients with bipolar disorder might be explained on the basis of
hyperactivity of neurons in the brain's limbic system, which modulates
people's experience and expression of emotion.

This approach to psychiatric reasoning is increasingly prevalent and
is consistent with Wilson's notion of consilience. The hunger for consilience in psychiatry is powerful and understandable. How is a psychiatrist supposed to be effective if he or she is working with an endless
and unconnected assemblage of ideas, theories, and concepts when trying to understand and treat a patient with manic symptoms? Is the
mania a psychological defense against unconsciously repressed sadness,
disappointment, or guilt? Was the manic episode precipitated by stress,
chaos, and disorder in the patient's home or workplace? Are there other
psychological or interpersonal factors in the patient's life that have
contributed to the manic state? These questions may be relevant, of
course, but they complicate the picture and may leave the patient and
clinician in a state of utter confusion and inaction. Conceptualizing the
clinical presentation as an intelligible and unified process that is rooted
in brain dysfunction may be a welcome relief to clinician and patient
alike. It may offer clarity and focus that allow them to take useful steps
toward managing the troubling symptoms, perhaps with psychotropic
medication.

But what if the neatly unified explanation leaves important clinical
factors out of the picture? Perhaps the patient has a genetic susceptibility to bipolar disorder (based on a family history of the condition), has
abnormalities on brain scans that might predispose to the disorder or
reveal an underlying neurological condition that mimics the disorder,
and would benefit from taking mood-stabilizing medications such as
lithium. However, perhaps the manic symptoms arise primarily when the
patient is suffering a blow to self-esteem, or is mourning an unbearably
painful loss, or is trying to avoid a daunting challenge at home or at
work. A convincing and useful explanation of the patient's bipolar disorder might require the introduction of a wide assortment of psychological and interpersonal concepts, including conscious and unconscious
motivation and communication. Likewise, if both biological and

psychosocial factors contribute to the patient's presentation, then the treatment of the disorder might be most effective if it encompasses a wide variety of therapeutic modalities, such as medications and talk therapy in combination.

As the psychiatrist approaches the patient with bipolar disorder, should he or she aim to achieve consilience or struggle to tolerate complexity and disorder? This question constitutes the central challenge to twenty-first century psychiatrists in their everyday practice. In a paper titled "Unity and Diversity in Psychiatry: Some Philosophical Issues," David Dewhurst and I. Patrick Burges Watson (1996) conceded that the scientific approach may allow psychiatrists to bring order to a confusing mess of clinical concepts, but argued primarily that mental disorders are so complex as to necessitate a "diversity of languages in psychiatry." On the other hand, in an article titled "Biological Psychiatry: Is There Any Other Kind?," psychiatrist Samuel Guze (1989) preferred the field's growing proclivity toward unifying psychiatric reasoning within the domain of empirical science. In an article titled "Science, Humanism, and the Nature of Medical Practice: A Phenomenological View," psychiatrist Michael Schwartz and philosopher Osborne Wiggins (1985) delineated the persistent tension between scientific order and human complexity in contemporary clinical work. Rather than advocating for either consilience or disorder in medicine and psychiatry, Schwartz and Wiggins turned their attention to the human "life world"—the realm of ordinary, day-to-day human experience—that precedes any scientific or clinical attempt to explain it or alter it via treatment.

These theorists and clinicians are not alone in their struggle to negotiate the science/humanism divide in clinical practice. The way psychiatrists choose to grapple with the consilience/disorder debate posed by philosophers of science will have profound effects on clinical practice in the twenty-first century. Tending toward Wilson's notion of consilience, some explanatory models in contemporary psychiatry are primarily scientific, whereas other models, which are more in keeping with Dupré's view of disorder and complexity, are primarily humanistic. The two approaches stand in a dialectical relationship to one another insofar as clinicians often move back and forth between science and humanism as they strive to synthesize the two approaches. Dialectical reasoning in psychiatry entails careful attention to both approaches and vigorous efforts to integrate them in a constructive way.

Intriguingly, one approach always seems to give way to the other approach in psychiatric practice—and this peculiarity is what makes psychiatric reasoning truly dialectical. As the psychiatrist describes clinical symptoms and locates the patient in a general diagnostic category, the patient as an individual begins to slip away—and the psychiatrist who recognizes the oversimplification will find a way to notice and take account of the patient's uniqueness. Conversely, the more a clinical psychiatrist tunes into a patient's unique human characteristics, the more he or she will experience an urge to compare and contrast the patient's experience with that of other people in similar circumstances or with similar disorders. Both processes—individuation and categorization of the patient—are entirely ordinary, and probably quite necessary, in clinical psychiatry. The dialectical process does not lead to the triumph of one approach over the other, but instead to a dynamic equilibrium between scientific and humanistic concepts, in which both poles of the dialectic play important roles in a broad-minded and inclusive treatment.

The way psychiatrists work through the dialectic of science and humanism has major scientific and ethical significance, insofar as it reflects what they deem valuable in rendering people's behavior intelligible and it leads them to treat their patients in particular ways. On the scientific side of the dialectic, we discover an impulse to explain human experience and behavior in accordance with concepts that are part and parcel of specialized theories, such as clinical neuroscience or cognitive-behavioral therapy (CBT). These theories tend to carefully define but also restrict what counts as a rigorous and useful explanatory concept. The clinical neuroscientist focuses on neurophysiological bases of behavior and explains abnormalities in thinking, emotion, and behavior on the basis of anatomical lesions or functional derangements in the brain. Thus, he or she may exclude from explanations such psychological factors as self-critical thinking and unconscious fantasies. On the other hand, when trying to account for psychiatric syndromes such as depression and anxiety, the cognitive-behavioral therapist concentrates on conscious mental processes (such as automatic, self-defeating thoughts) and repetitive, pathogenic patterns of behavior. In so doing, the cognitive-behavioral therapist may give short shrift to important biological factors, such as neurotransmitter functioning and psychopharmacological activity.

The reduction and elimination of certain explanatory constructs, and the development of (and clear emphasis on) others, represent both the strength and the weakness of the scientific side of the science/humanism divide. Specialized scientific models and theories, which may be conceptually elegant and clinically useful, are often a welcome result. Scientific methodology in psychiatry has led to astonishing advances. There is a clear rationale for scientific reductionism in the setting of neuropsychiatric disorders like Huntington's disease, a debilitating and ultimately fatal illness characterized by abnormal, involuntary movements, major depression, and progressive dementia. The onset of Huntington's disease, which usually strikes men in early to middle adulthood, can be predicted and explained entirely on the basis of an inherited genetic anomaly. Unfortunately, despite the remarkable elucidation of the cause of Huntington's disease, no treatment has been found for it and the disease remains fatal. Most psychiatric illnesses cannot yet be explained in such a unitary fashion as Huntington's disease, with its clear and indisputable genetic cause. However, psychiatric researchers are actively conducting promising investigations into the genetic variations that predispose to major depression and other mental disorders. Placebo-controlled trials of psychotropic medications have enhanced the treatment of numerous psychiatric disorders (such as major depression, bipolar disorder, and schizophrenia) and well-designed empirical studies of psychosocial interventions (such as CBT) also have demonstrated therapeutic efficacy for these conditions.

The move toward reductive explanation in natural science in general, and in human sciences like psychiatry in particular, arguably is a dominant trend in recent years. In *Consilience: The Unity of Knowledge*, Wilson (1998, 105) asserted that "belief in the intrinsic unity of knowledge rides ultimately on the hypothesis that every mental process has a physical grounding and is consistent with the natural sciences." Psychiatrist Abraham Rudnick (2002) argued that the past half-century has seen a "molecular turn" in psychiatry toward a "neurotransmitter dysfunction paradigm" of mental illness. Along these lines, the power of brain science and psychopharmacology to explain and alter behavior appears to support reductive materialism—the theory that neuroscience can account for all human behavior and that psychological concepts can be reduced by "bridge laws" to biological concepts that are more generalized and verifiable. Diagnostic and therapeutic successes of biological psychiatry attest to the robustness of such bridge laws and the rationale for reducing mental concepts to neurological ones. Twentieth-century psychiatry showed that numerous disorders that used to be explained psychologically could be better explained biologically, as the result of genetic anomalies, strokes, brain tumors, endocrine diseases, infections, seizures, neuronal degeneration, and other alterations in brain functioning. This notion prompted psychoanalyst Robert Wallerstein (1994, xi) to reflect that there is now a widespread belief that an "enhanced knowledge of the biological dimensions of mental disorders renders psychosocial and psychological approaches far less relevant—if not completely obsolete."

Nevertheless, biological explanatory models in psychiatry may go too far in emphasizing the primacy of just one type of explanation and treatment. Large-scale clinical studies of the treatment of major depression (e.g., Keller et al. 2000)—which compare the efficacy of psychotherapy alone, antidepressant medication alone, and combined treatment—have suggested clear benefits of combining psychological and biological approaches. The benefit of integrating psychotherapy and psychopharmacology to treat depression and other psychiatric disorders flies in the face of strict reductive materialism. Emerging biological models of depression have provided a foundation for the development of powerful treatments with antidepressant medications and electroconvulsive therapy (both of which are now well-established treatment modalities) and with novel techniques such as transcranial magnetic stimulation and vagal nerve stimulation (both of which are still in an experimental phase). These scientific models in themselves, however, are inadequate to explain or treat complex clinical phenomena in many cases. Clinical vignettes presented in chapter 3 and elsewhere throughout this book will help to highlight this point and support the critical role of multimodal therapeutic approaches that carefully combine biological and psychotherapeutic elements.

Of course, reductive explanatory models can emerge from either end of the mind/brain spectrum. At the psychological extreme, for example, psychiatrists at the Chestnut Lodge in the late 1980s unsuccessfully treated a patient's major depression with psychoanalytic therapy alone, and accepted an explanatory model that unwisely overlooked the relevance of brain chemistry and pharmacology. The patient, Rafael Osheroff, recovered when he was finally treated with psychotropic medications at another facility; he later sued Chestnut Lodge for negligence and sparked significant controversy around the issue of a patient's right to effective treatment (Klerman 1990; Stone 1990). There is broad agreement now that psychoanalytic psychotherapy alone is inadequate to treat most cases of severe depression. Thus, antidepressant medications and electroconvulsive therapy have become key parts of the current standard of care. There is no doubt that reductive psychologism can be just as rigid and restrictive, and thus inimical to effective and ethically grounded patient care, as reductive materialism.

Reductionism of either the biological or the psychological variety calls to mind the adage that if one's only tool is a hammer, everything can begin to look like a nail. Patients may be short-changed by hard-nosed and inflexible diagnostic and therapeutic approaches that are reductionistic in either the biological or the psychological direction. In many clinical situations, patients are not served well by rigid adherence to scientific theories that emphasize certain explanatory constructs but exclude others that may be equally essential to their recovery. Good clinical care often depends on an "idiographic" approach that views the patient as an individual agent with unique traits and circumstances, rather than on a "nomothetic" approach that strives to place the patient on a procrustean bed of rigid science (Schafer 1999). However, if the idiographic approach does not ground itself in plausible empirical evidence, it runs the risk of fuzzy-minded reasoning and truth may suffer—along with patients and the overall respectability of psychiatry as a rigorous medical science.

When working on the scientific side of the science/humanism divide, the psychiatrist aims to practice evidence-based medicine and employ a well-demarcated set of explanatory concepts to achieve unified, empirically supported accounts of human behavior. But exclusion of alternative explanatory concepts may be detrimental, especially when explaining multifaceted behavior and treating individuals whose emotions are conflicted and whose behavior is maladaptive. Narrowly focused, scientific explanatory models in psychiatry may be flawed and inadequate insofar as they restrict the clinician's flexibility in making diagnoses and implementing treatments. If a psychiatrist applies an empirically validated, evidence-based approach in a rigid or mechanized way (perhaps according to "practice guidelines" established by experts in the field), the patient may benefit (perhaps in the form of symptomatic relief) but also feel that meaningful aspects of his or her existence (such as inner experiences of grief, shame, joy, or spirituality) were overlooked or neglected. The clinical benefit may be incomplete because some important intrapsychic and interpersonal contributors to the patient's suffering have not been addressed. Some psychiatrists in recent years have observed that "too great an emphasis on evidence-based medicine oversimplifies the complex and interpersonal nature of clinical care" (Williams and Garner 2002, 8).

Human action and experience are usually too complex to be captured adequately in explanations that appeal only to the concepts and tools of a single discipline on the scientific side of the science/humanism dialectic. So it is not surprising to discover another side of the dialectic—the humanistic side—that is equally compelling and problematic. Here we find an impulse toward explanatory diversity and recognition of the complex nature of human existence. Humanistic approaches hold the appeal of acknowledging the multifactorial causation of most mental disorders and the irreducible, subjective experience of suffering with such a disorder. In the book *Approaches to the Mind: Movement of the Psychiatric Schools from Sects toward Science*, psychiatrist Leston Havens (1973) described an empirical-scientific ("objective-descriptive") approach to psychiatric explanation and contrasted it with three humanistic approaches: the psychoanalytic, the existential, and the interpersonal. These latter three approaches employ various forms of psychotherapy and rely on the clinician's attempts to understand and work with the patient's psychological conflicts, subjective experiences, and social interactions.

Psychiatric eclecticism is one manifestation of the humanistic impulse toward open-mindedness and diversity in clinical explanation and treatment. Psychiatrist Joel Yager (1977, 739) described what he called the psychiatrist's "eclectic mental operation" as the attempt to "view a situation through each of several frames of reference." Especially in complex and treatment-refractory cases, Yager argued, psychiatrists need to have "either the cognitive flexibility to shift perspective or sufficient knowledge about alternative frames of reference or alternative treatment skills." When confronted with the challenge of treating a patient with mania, for example, the eclectic psychiatrist would have to consider biological vulnerabilities and the role of medications, intrapsychic factors and the role of psychotherapy, and the social context and possible need to help the patient organize and structure his or her day-to-day existence. The eclectic psychiatrist appreciates Dupré's "disorder of things" when it comes to explaining the multiple human factors that contribute to the patient's presentation. On this humanistic side of the dialectic, the clinician has a broad and unrestricted set of tools with which to explain why people act as they do, and to integrate seemingly different tools in order to treat patients sensitively and effectively.

Humanistic approaches acknowledge the complexity of psychological motivation, existential experience, interpersonal relationships, and sociocultural determinants of the mind. They recognize as well that human values and ethical considerations cannot be excluded from diagnostic and treatment methodologies in psychiatry, regardless of how scientifically or technologically advanced those methodologies become. But many humanistic models also are incomplete because they tend to be subjective and to lack a well-defined empirical basis. If applied in a careless or uncritical fashion, these models can be vague and lack sufficient rigor. Eclecticism, by using any and all of the approaches in psychiatry, may lose sight of the power and the efficacy of a specific approach to particular cases. It may cause diagnostic formulations and treatment plans to become unnecessarily complicated and unfocused, when concentration on a particular, highly focused approach would have sufficed. Eclecticism has been roundly criticized for failing to discern when to implement a specific explanatory model and for its tendency to "underplay differences" and "homogenize complexities" in clinical explanation (Havens 1973).

Another approach on the humanistic side of the science/humanism dialectic is the biopsychosocial model, which was first described by

George Engel (1977, 1980) as an alternative to the reductive explanatory models that dominated medicine and psychiatry. The biopsychosocial model assigns equal weight to the entire gamut of explanatory concepts that are relevant to psychiatry, including natural science, individual psychology, social interactions, and organizational factors as studied in economics, politics, sociology, and anthropology. The model aims to describe phenomena at each of these levels of explanation, and it suggests that causal explanations of mental disorders ought to incorporate any concept that impinges on human lives. In the case of bipolar disorder, for example, the mood swings from depression to mania would need to be understood at the level of the gene, intracellular processes, brain neurochemistry, individual psychology (such as personality traits and unconscious motivations), and social factors such as the family, the school, the workplace, financial conditions, and other aspects of the situation in which the patient's life is embedded. The biopsychosocial model is helpful insofar as it calls the clinician's attention to both the relevant science of human behavior and the humanistic complexity of the person seeking mental health care. But like eclecticism, it has been criticized for encouraging clinicians to assemble many "lumps of data" but providing little guidance as to which data are most relevant to a particular case and how those data can be ordered into a coherent relation to one another (McLaren 1998). By failing to provide such guidance, the biopsychosocial model can leave the clinical psychiatrist in a state of confusion about what to do with a vast and chaotic array of theories, concepts, and clinical data.

When carried to an extreme, humanistic approaches can degenerate into a relativistic or "postmodern" approach to psychiatry, in which the validity of all empirical study of human behavior is fundamentally called into question. There has been significant debate recently about the implications of postmodernism—a theory that rejects the possibility of acquiring objective knowledge and espouses the context-dependent features of all human understanding—for psychiatry and psychoanalysis (Lewis 2000; Holt 2002). Some postmodern thinkers have gone so far as to argue that biomedical science is irrelevant to clinical psychiatry. In the article "Postpsychiatry: A New Direction for Mental Health," psychiatrists Patrick Bracken and Philip Thomas (2001, 725) argued against modern psychiatrists' impulse to "replace spiritual, moral, political, and folk understandings of madness with the technological framework of psychopathology and neuroscience." They suggested, instead, that empirical evidence in clinical psychiatry is context-bound and value-driven, and thus that psychiatric theory does not rise to the level of the "neutral, objective, and disinterested."

This stance prompted Bracken and Thomas to advocate a "hermeneutic" approach to psychiatry, which focuses on narrative, experiential, and interpersonal dimensions of mental suffering. Hermeneutic psychiatrists believe that mental disorders are socially constructed entities that reflect personal and societal values; therefore, they reject the idea that these disorders can be defined on an objective and empirically derived basis. The hermeneutic approach, unfortunately, neglects helpful scientific dimensions of psychiatry, such as well-established associations between certain brain lesions and mental disorders. The biopsychosocial model, eclecticism, postmodern psychiatry, and hermeneutics are appropriately sensitive to the full range of humanistic factors in psychiatry, but they run the risk of overlooking the fact that, in some situations, psychiatrists can identify a specific, evidence-based cause of the disorder and can recommend appropriately tailored treatment on that basis.

Humanistic approaches to psychiatry do not necessarily have these flaws. There has been a gathering movement in the behavioral sciences in recent years to bring humanistic approaches under the microscope of scientific observation and method. While most humanistic models in psychiatry highlight personal meaning and subjective experience (and consign empirical observation to a secondary status or to complete irrelevance), there have been admirable but problematic attempts to render various humanistic approaches to psychiatry more scientific. Psychologist Drew Westen and colleagues (2004) described the science/humanism split in contemporary psychotherapy: some therapists believe that any particular form of psychotherapy should be offered to patients (and be reimbursed by their insurance companies) if and only if it has been validated in empirical studies, while other therapists believe most patients only benefit from an unconstrained type of psychotherapy that flexibly integrates diverse approaches, such as a mixture of psychodynamic and cognitive-behavioral tools. In an article by Benedict Carey in the *New York Times* on August 10, 2004 ("For Psychotherapy's Claims, Skeptics Demand Proof"), the science/humanism split in the field was described as a modern-day "civil war" with many people not "in the mood for healing" on either side of the debate. "On one side are experts who argue that what therapists do in their consulting rooms should be backed by scientific studies proving its worth," Carey wrote. "On the other side are those who say that the push for this evidence threatens the very things that make psychotherapy work in the first place."

The empirical studies in question are designed to assess the process and outcome of psychotherapy. Psychiatrist Norman Doidge (1997) and Westen and colleagues (2004) published articles that review some of the most important psychotherapy-outcome studies conducted in recent years. They have described the ideal characteristics of a rigorous empirical study of this kind: evaluation of patients with a single diagnosis; presence of a comparison (control) group that receives no treatment; assessment of well-defined symptoms; use of a standardized treatment manual; participation of highly experienced clinicians; and use of raters of clinical outcomes who are blind as to whether a given patient was in the experimental group or the comparison group. Although no study to date has met all these rigorous criteria, Doidge noted that a handful of reasonably sound studies conducted in recent decades revealed a 60 to 90 percent success rate for patients who received psychoanalysis or dynamic psychotherapy. The most sophisticated of these studies was a prospective trial that followed forty-two patients in psychoanalytic treatment at the Menninger Clinic in Topeka, Kansas, between 1954 and 1984. Although a substantial number of the subjects had more severe psychological problems than patients in psychoanalytic therapy today, 23 percent of them still showed moderate improvement and 36 percent made very good improvement according to the outcome ratings. The trial was limited by the use of student clinicians, a relatively small number of subjects, and the absence of a comparison group—which, of course, would have been impractical to establish and maintain for thirty years. In spite of these limitations, this study (and others like it) showed that the efficacy of humanistic therapies like psychoanalysis can be assessed empirically—and that they merit further study based on preliminary evidence that they are remarkably effective.

While scientific studies of humanistic approaches to psychiatry may be feasible and desirable, it is important to balance this consideration with honest recognition of the fact that such studies inevitably have flaws and limitations. In most well-conducted medication trials in psychiatry, there are an experimental group and a comparison group, and the clinician and the patient both are blind as to whether the active drug or a placebo is being administered. This is impossible to achieve in psychotherapy studies, where the nature of the treatment is patently obvious to clinician and patient alike. Other unavoidable flaws of psychotherapy-outcome studies are that in the real world the therapist is selected by the patient (rather than being assigned by a researcher) and that the frequency of sessions, as well as the overall length of treatment, is flexibly adapted to the patient's needs rather than preestablished in a research protocol. Humanistic treatments in psychiatry, which focus on the patient's subjective experiences and individualized needs, inevitably sacrifice some scientific rigor because they cannot be easily validated empirically; and when they are studied empirically, the research findings usually cannot be generalized consistently or reliably. Despite recent efforts to place humanistic approaches to psychiatry under the lens of scientific scrutiny and study, these approaches retain a fundamental basis in the mysteries, complexities, and existential dimensions of human experience.

While empirical science suggests that some humanistic approaches to psychiatry are likely to be effective, there are some clinical situations that require a single conceptual approach. At times complex human behavior can and should be explained and treated with a delimited set of scientific concepts. A temporal lobe seizure disorder or a metabolic disorder with psychological effects may explain (and suggest the appropriate treatment for) an elaborate set of abnormal behaviors; psychodynamic or hermeneutic concepts may be much less important, or beside the point, in such neuropsychiatric cases. Conversely, brain science may be largely irrelevant to the formulation and treatment of other cases, such as those in which the root causes and clinical manifestations of the patient's difficulties appear to reside in personality traits, interpersonal relationships, and family dynamics. In a paper on the relations among four major conceptual approaches in psychiatry (medical, psychological, behavioral, and social), psychiatrist Aaron Lazare (1973, 350) wrote that in most situations "a psychiatrist will employ several conceptual models with the knowledge that all reflect some aspect of truth but all are incomplete versions of truth"; however, Lazare pointed out that "in limited cases a single conceptual model will suffice to explain the disorder and provide treatment."

Lazare highlighted the notion that scientific reductionism and humanistic eclecticism both have a place in clinical psychiatry. Practicing psychiatrists find themselves caught in a conceptual tension between reductionism and eclecticism, and often are tempted to move toward one approach or the other. The scientific side of the dialectic calls the clinical psychiatrist's attention to relevant empirical understanding and evidence-based treatments of mental disorders, but it tends to reduce the range of options for making diagnostic formulations and therapeutic paradigm choices. The humanistic side of the dialectic, meanwhile, calls the clinician's attention to the complexities and subjective features of psychiatric disorders, but it lacks a clear, consistent, and rigorous theoretical basis. There is a profound need, therefore, to critique current explanatory paradigms and develop alternative paradigms that are sensitive to the opposing impulses toward science and humanism. At this time, unfortunately, there is no well-defined and widely accepted third option that navigates between both sides of the science/humanism divide. In fact, forces in contemporary science (and in society in general) tend to favor one side of the divide over the other. As Luhrmann demonstrated in *Of Two Minds: The Growing Disorder in American Psychiatry*, the discipline is polarized into biomedical and psychodynamic camps—often to the detriment of patient care, research, and training of future clinicians.

Twenty-first-century psychiatrists must acknowledge the complexity and irreducibility of mental illnesses but at the same time strive for scientific rigor in their clinical practice and their academic research. Conversely, they must keep in mind that patients may be harmed by hard-nosed and inflexible diagnostic and therapeutic approaches, even if those approaches are evidence-based. In many clinical situations, patients are not served well by rigid adherence to theories that emphasize certain well-validated explanatory constructs but exclude others that may be equally essential. How are contemporary clinical psychiatrists to use the strengths and to minimize the shortcomings of both sides of the divide between science and humanism? The nature of mental health care, research, and education in the twenty-first century will depend on how psychiatrists frame this question and struggle to answer it. If psychiatrists are not equipped to employ dialectical reasoning to heal the theoretical and clinical wounds that have resulted from their dividing the person into an object of scientific scrutiny and a subject of personal experience, they may not be able to formulate their cases comprehensively or to provide patients with the benefits of ethical and cutting-edge care. Moreover, they may not be able to synthesize disparate conceptual approaches to generate new understanding of mental suffering or to educate future psychiatric clinicians and researchers in the art and science of the field.

Psychiatry is a special discipline in part because of its equal recognition and use of empirical science and humanistic values. Some disciplines, such as molecular biology and physics, essentially can make do with the empirical approach alone. On the other hand, some fields, such as literary and feminist studies, focus primarily on human values and the nature of subjective experience. But psychiatrists have no such option: at all times they face the challenge of integrating scientific and humanistic approaches so that the whole person is recognized and cared for. Healing the conceptual wounds in contemporary psychiatry is not simply an abstract task, but an urgent ethical imperative on which rigorous and humane clinical care, research, and training depend. It is, therefore, of the utmost importance to define practical and theoretical approaches to bridge the science/humanism divide in psychiatric practice, research, and education. Psychiatrists must recognize the complexity and irreducibility of human mental suffering but at the same time strive for scientific rigor in their clinical practice, academic research, and efforts to train a new generation of practitioners.

Chapter 2 presents a clinical sensibility and methodology that aim to achieve these goals. The approach it will delineate, which is grounded in classical American pragmatism and contemporary pragmatic bioethics, employs dialectical reasoning to work through the science/humanism divide in psychiatry. It furnishes an opportunity for twenty-first-century psychiatrists to heal the conceptual wounds that have resulted from the longstanding tendency to split the patient into an objective specimen for scientific study and a complex human subject whose behavior is meaningful and whose personal experience evokes wonder, empathy, compassion, and respect.

2

A Pragmatic Approach to Psychiatry

The scientific and humanistic sides of the explanatory dialectic in clinical psychiatry both have their merits and shortcomings. Is it possible to develop a conceptually sound model of human behavior that might serve as a theoretical basis for psychiatry, and that would successfully integrate psychiatric science and humanism? We can begin to approach this question by considering some ideas from contemporary philosophy of science. Philosopher Robert McCauley (1996) described how explanatory systems that are distinct but deal with the same phenomena—such as psychology and neuroscience as applied to human behavior—can co-evolve. In his "co-evolution$_s$" model—where the subscript stands for scientific revolutions—competing theories become so incompatible that one of them must be reduced or eliminated by the other. This is the coevolutionary theory favored by Wilson and others who espouse reductive materialism. An alternative model is McCauley's "co-evolution$_p$"— where the subscript stands for pluralism—in which a diverse set of concepts are understood as compatible and can provide greater explanatory resources. Such a pluralistic mode of explanation, provided that it is rigorous and heeds relevant empirical evidence, might provide psychiatrists with the flexibility they require to integrate scientific and humanistic approaches as clinically indicated.

Where might we turn to discover the basis of an explanatory model for psychiatry that is pluralistic, rigorous, and focused on everyday clinical needs? I believe that philosophical pragmatism—a form of reasoning that focuses on achieving practical outcomes rather than defining abstract theories—can provide a helpful set of principles and tools by which psychiatrists could work through the science/humanism divide that continues to bedevil clinical psychiatry. There is burgeoning interest in the history and theoretical basis of classical American pragmatism as developed in the late nineteenth and early twentieth centuries by such thinkers as Charles Sanders Peirce, William James, and John Dewey (Diggins 1994; Dickstein 1998; Rosenthal, Hausman, and Anderson 1999; Rescher 2000). The American pragmatists were a diverse and informally connected group of intellectuals who developed what John Smith, a philosopher and scholar of philosophical pragmatism, called an "indigenous American philosophy" in his introduction to the volume *Classical American Pragmatism: Its Contemporary Vitality* (1999). The American pragmatists struggled to develop ideas and patterns of thought that were relevant to the multifarious challenges of a growing nation, such as building new towns and cities, providing public education, ensuring representative government, and establishing civic institutions that included people of different races and religious backgrounds. Facing these concrete, practical challenges of day-to-day life, it is not surprising that the American pragmatists were eager to cast off the conceptual shackles of certain distinctively European systems of thought such as Immanuel Kant's philosophy, with its focus on immutable characteristics of the human mind and on absolute moral laws.

Instead, the American pragmatists offered many novel and open-minded suggestions on how to think about the entire gamut of human activities, such as ethics and religion, politics and government, mathematics and science, education and social life. In the book *The Metaphysical Club: A Story of Ideas in America* (2001), Louis Menand brilliantly traced the historical and philosophical origins of American pragmatism to the mid-nineteenth century and the Civil War, which challenged those who survived it to articulate a more modern set of ideas that could help to maintain civil order and allow Americans to adapt to a whole new set of social conditions brought about by the end of slavery, the beginning of the industrial revolution, the expansion of the nation westward, and other upheavals in American life. The American pragmatists aimed to distance themselves not only from the abstract ideologies of European philosophers, but also from the assumptions and prejudices that characterized prewar American life in the North and the South. As they did so, they were deeply influenced by Charles Darwin's theory of evolution (as delineated in *On the Origin of Species* in 1859), which brought to the intellectual foreground important ideas about change, variation, and adaptation to novel circumstances. Peirce, James, and Dewey employed different modes of inquiry in their respective disciplines but, as Menand (2001, xi–xii) pointed out, they shared a common attitude:

They all believed that ideas are not "out there" waiting to be discovered, but are tools—like forks and knives and microchips—that people devise to cope with the world in which they find themselves. They believed that ideas are produced not by individuals, but by groups of individuals—that ideas are social. They believed that ideas do not develop according to some inner logic of their own, but are entirely dependent, like germs, on their human carriers and the environment. And they believed that since ideas are provisional responses to particular and unreproducible circumstances, their survival depends not on their immutability but on their adaptability.

The American pragmatists arrived at this basic orientation from their work in several different domains. Charles Sanders Peirce (1839–1914) was a child prodigy who became a wide-ranging intellectual at Harvard with strong aptitudes for mathematics, logic, astronomy, and philosophical argumentation. In the early 1870s, Peirce, James, and several others (including Oliver Wendell Holmes Jr. and Chauncey Wright) formed a discussion group in Cambridge—which Peirce would later refer to as "The Metaphysical Club"—in which they discussed ideas that laid the foundation for the work on philosophical pragmatism that followed during the ensuing decades. Menand recounted the engaging idiosyncrasies of Peirce's character and the dramatic course of events that led to his removal from the Harvard faculty in the 1870s and from the Johns Hopkins University faculty years later—and the pariah status that Peirce maintained thereafter. Nonetheless, even without a prestigious university appointment, Peirce's intellectual influence continued unabated into the opening years of the twentieth century. With a deep faith in the power of science, Peirce argued that careful observation and ongoing empirical testing by a community of scientists ultimately could lead to coherent findings and useful knowledge about the natural world. At the same time, Peirce cautioned that scientific observations are fallible and inexact, that they always must remain open to further testing and revision, and that their accuracy or truth must be assessed in terms of their practical utility.

William James (1842–1910) graduated from Harvard Medical School in 1869, but never actually practiced or taught clinical medicine. He briefly taught physiology after he graduated from medical school and recovered from a severe episode of depression, and he then moved into experimental psychology and later to academic philosophy. His interest in and commitment to science and humanism are reflected in the fact that he published one of the most important works ever in experimental psychology in 1890 (*The Principles of Psychology*) and, in 1901–1902, delivered an ambitious set of lectures on the diversity of spirituality and religion as practiced throughout the world (*The Varieties of Religious Experience*). But James never developed an inflexible allegiance to a particular school of thought. He was an extraordinarily open-minded, far-reaching thinker whose philosophical work and public persona were equally renowned by the 1890s. At that time he had begun to lecture and to write on the merits of philosophical pragmatism and he promoted the widespread use of the term *pragmatism*, which Peirce had coined during the days they spent together in the metaphysical club in 1872. In writings from the 1890s and the early 1900s, James described pragmatism as a method of thought and scientific investigation that aims for favorable practical consequences for people in ordinary life, that recognizes the fallibility of empirical observations, and that always incorporates a plurality of factors that shape human existence.

At the age of 35, John Dewey (1859–1952) was appointed chair of the philosophy department at the University of Chicago, where he solidified his lifelong commitment to education. Dewey founded the Laboratory School (which exists in Chicago to this day) on the basis of the pragmatic principles of pedagogy he helped to define. Believing that knowing and doing were inseparable, Dewey instituted a curriculum that used goal-directed and collaborative activities (such as cooking) to teach students such traditionally abstract subjects as arithmetic and chemistry. In 1904, Dewey moved to Columbia University's Teachers College, where he spent the remainder of his long career. By then, pragmatism already had emerged as a major philosophical movement and Dewey became one of its most influential advocates. In philosophical papers he wrote during the ensuing years, Dewey advanced the core pragmatic argument that ideas must be assessed on the basis of their capacity to help people cope with the challenges of their everyday lives. Like James, he was deeply skeptical that philosophy or empirical science could lead to absolute, objective, or immutable truth; he criticized this traditional scientific impulse in his 1929 lecture "The Quest for Certainty: A Study of the Relation of Knowledge and Action." Dewey's pragmatic approach depended on flexible and open-minded habits of thinking among a community of inquirers. He believed that multiple forms of intellectual inquiry were relevant for diverse goals and that each form of inquiry had to develop its own methodological standards based on its subject matter and its aim. He argued as well that scientific inquiry always occurs in a social context that shapes the nature of the results and the uses to which they are put.

For the purposes of this chapter, it will be useful to draw on the work of Peirce, James, and Dewey to identify four separate but closely related organizing principles of classical American pragmatism. Here and throughout the book, I will refer to these fundamental principles of philosophical pragmatism as the four *p*'s. They include (1) the *practical* dimensions of all scientific inquiry; (2) the *pluralistic* nature of the phenomena studied by science and the tools that are used to study those phenomena; (3) the *participatory* role of many individuals with different perspectives in the necessarily interpersonal process of scientific inquiry; and (4) the *provisional* and flexible character of scientific explanation. The four *p*'s reflect the fact that Peirce, James, and Dewey believed deeply in the promise of the scientific enterprise but cautioned that science always must be understood in its human context, which is messy, complicated, and constantly evolving in unforeseen ways. With this point in mind, let us consider each of the four *p*'s in turn and then examine their roles in transcending the science/humanism divide in contemporary medicine and psychiatry.

As to the first *p*, a core belief shared by each of the classical American pragmatists (and applicable to clinical psychiatry today) was that the fundamental aim of empirical science and other quests for knowledge ought to be favorable practical outcomes for people in ordinary life. Abstract philosophical or scientific knowledge, according to their worldview, was either unobtainable or irrelevant to achieving the most important goals of everyday life. Theories are not developed for their own sake but rather to be employed instrumentally, in the service of a human good or everyday challenge. In "A Definition of Pragmatism" (1904), Peirce wrote that the pragmatic analysis of any given concept was the attempt to trace "the conceivable practical consequences . . . of the affirmation or denial of the concept." In "The Need for a Recovery of Philosophy" (1917), Dewey argued that philosophy and science are results-oriented pursuits that necessarily occur within a social matrix and that "philosophy shall develop ideas relevant to the actual crises of life, ideas influential in dealing with them and tested by the assistance they afford." In "What Pragmatism Means" (1907, 142), James outlined the pragmatic approach as follows:

The pragmatic method is primarily a method of settling metaphysical disputes that otherwise might be interminable. Is the world one or many?—fated or free?—material or spiritual?—here are notions either of which may or may not hold good of the world; and disputes over such notions are unending. The pragmatic method in such cases is to try to interpret each notion by tracing its respective practical consequences. . . . Whenever a dispute is serious, we ought to be able to show some practical difference that must follow from one side or the other's being right.

As to the second p, classical American pragmatism also highlighted the diverse elements of scientific explanation. In *A Pluralistic Universe*, published in 1909, James argued that the pragmatic scientist aims to organize empirical knowledge into a unified, coherent system of thought, but always entertains the possibility of "a pluralistic and incompletely integrated universe" (p. 106). In his 1906 lecture "The One and The Many," James similarly argued that "acquaintance with reality's diversities is as important as understanding their connexion" (p. 65). Like the multiplicity of religious beliefs and practices he cataloged in *The Varieties of Religious Experience*, scientific pluralism (the second p) was a given for James; there are many natural and human phenomena in the world that deserve study, and they exist side by side with one another. James believed there is no way to tether them to a single conceptual foundation as suggested by Wilson's philosophy of consilience. Thus, James explicitly rejected Hegel's "monism," the theory that complex elements of the universe can be understood in a unitary fashion. What James retained of Hegel's early-nineteenth-century philosophy, however, was a methodology based on dialectical reasoning—where one approach necessarily gives way to an opposing approach and where two (or more) of the approaches end up coevolving in a dynamic equilibrium. "There is a dialectic movement in things," James wrote in *A Pluralistic Universe*, "but it is one that can be described and accounted for in terms of the pluralistic vision of things far more naturally than in the monistic terms to which Hegel finally reduced it" (p. 90).

In addition, the American pragmatists suggested that truth is the outcome of a process that is participatory (the third *p*) and that aims at identifying what works in any given situation. In a pluralistic society, opposing viewpoints are inevitable and conflict must be managed in a civil and constructive fashion. In an essay titled "Pragmatism, Pluralism, and the Healing of Wounds," philosopher Richard J. Bernstein (1988) argued that the American pragmatists advocated a "dialogical response" to pluralism and conflict whereby opposing individuals, after they have debated a conflict, move toward mutual understanding—or, at the very least, respectfully agree to disagree. The same methodological principles apply to the scientific process. Different scientists may approach the same natural phenomena with different background assumptions and methods of inquiry. They either replicate each other's findings or call those findings into question, thereby prompting further study and dialogue. A pluralistic set of perspectives hopefully leads to a better understanding of the world at some point.

However, as Menand (2001) explained, the American pragmatists differed in their views about how this pluralism could foster greater understanding. Peirce tended to believe that multiple inquiries and observations ultimately can converge on genuine understanding; in contrast, James and Dewey tended to be skeptical that science could ever achieve such a level of certainty. As a result, Peirce distanced himself in the early 1900s from James's skepticism about the capabilities of empirical science. Instead, Peirce suggested that James had hijacked the term *pragmatism*, and so he decided to name his more optimistic sensibility about empirical science *pragmaticism*. But the less cumbersome term *pragmatism* had already achieved widespread popularity and to this day remains associated with the works of Peirce, James, and Dewey alike.

In reality, though, Peirce, James, and Dewey were not so far from each other conceptually; each of them captured relevant dimensions of the scientific process. At times they all emphasized empirical science's promise and at other times they urged caution about its limitations and fallibilities. This is where the fourth *p* of classical American pragmatism—the provisional nature of scientific explanation—comes into play. Peirce, James, and Dewey advocated the concept of "fallibilism," which holds that objective truth is not readily available, that human knowledge is imbued with uncertainty, and that all scientific hypotheses must be rigorously and continually tested. A corollary of this view is that the empirical sciences (as well as the clinical sciences) are open-ended and evolving enterprises that require their practitioners to have a flexible, open-minded, and provisional sensibility. In his essay "A Guess at the Riddle" (1890), Peirce argued that scientific laws could be developed out of the "pure chance, irregularity, and indeterminacy" (p. 50) observed in natural events but that the laws on which scientific inquirers converge are imperfect and vulnerable to "aberrancy" (p. 51). Similarly, recognizing the pluralistic and evolving nature of human life and the natural world, James argued in his essay *Humanism and Truth* (1904) that "owing to the fact that all experience is a process, no point of view can ever be *the* last one" (p. 221). Dewey, emphasizing the open-ended and innovative nature of science, wrote in *The Need for a Recovery of Philosophy* (1917) that "a pragmatic intelligence is a creative intelligence, not a routine mechanic" (p. 67).

How can classical American pragmatism be applied to medicine and psychiatry in our own day? Can the four *p*'s as I have defined them help to guide clinical practice? The emergence in recent years of a pragmatic bioethics movement has suggested that the principles of Peirce, James, and Dewey can be usefully applied to problems that plague the individual doctor-patient relationship and the health-care system as a whole in an era that is remarkable for advancing medical technology, but also for uncertainty about how to apply that technology humanely and for a scarcity of financial resources to deliver it to large sectors of the nation's and world's population. An edited volume titled *Pragmatic Bioethics* (McGee 2003), a special issue of the *Journal of Medicine and Philosophy* that was devoted to pragmatism and bioethics (Arras 2003; Bellantoni 2003; Brendel 2003; Cooke 2003; Hester 2003; Schmidt-Felzmann 2003; Tollefsen and Cherry 2003; Trotter 2003), and related works (e.g., Miller, Fins, and Bachetta 1996; Hart 2002) demonstrate the relevance of philosophical pragmatism in contemporary medical settings. These endeavors in pragmatic bioethics apply the principles of classical American pragmatism to the dilemmas and challenges that physicians face in their everyday medical practice.

There is a fundamental belief among pragmatic bioethicists that the first *p*—the practical nature of scientific inquiry—needs to guide physicians as they provide clinical care. Medical ethics cannot depend on philosophical abstractions but ought to be engaged with the very real problems that emerge in the course of clinical practice. This view of medical ethics requires pragmatic reasoning. But if it is performed carelessly, pragmatic reasoning can run the risk of trading what is true for what happens to be expedient at a particular moment. This danger is well described by bioethicists who write on pragmatism. In the article "What Would John Dewey Do? The Promises and Perils of Pragmatic Bioethics," philosopher Christopher Tollefsen (2000) depicted the dangers of holding something to be true just because it happens to work (he considered James's reflections on whether a counterfeit banknote is valid simply because it has not yet been detected and is accepted as real currency). In modern medical science, the peril of pragmatism might involve believing that we have identified the underlying cause of a disease simply because we have found an effective treatment for it. Can we claim, for example, that major depression is caused by low levels of neurotransmitters (such as serotonin) in the brain just because medications that enhance serotonin levels have antidepressant effects? Or is the cause of depression more complex than that—and might the fact that antidepressant medications enhance serotonin levels be a red herring?

Some contemporary "neopragmatists," such as the philosopher Richard Rorty (1979, 1982), downplay the relevance of scientific realism and argue that a claim should be judged solely on the basis of its practical effects. A neopragmatic physician who, like Rorty, downplays empirical reality might accept too readily that what works in the clinic accurately reflects something about human biology. In addition to being intellectually unsatisfying, this distinctly postmodern form of reasoning is dangerous because it could threaten to shut down further inquiry into causes and novel therapies of some diseases. Pragmatic physicians who work in the tradition of Peirce, James, and Dewey aim to avoid this danger by committing themselves to scientific realism and openness to empirical testing of their beliefs. They keep in mind that new medical knowledge ought to be pursued (and is likely to emerge) and that the validity of their theories should not be equated with what happens to work best at any particular moment. Along these lines, psychologist Peter Zachar (2000, 170), a strong proponent of pragmatism in behavioral science, wrote that the pragmatist's openness to evolution of their models "cautions them from too easily believing that their categories directly correspond to how things really are." At the same time, the pragmatic clinician needs to make do with the current state of understanding and take action to help the patient achieve practical goals in the present.

With regard to the second *p* (pluralism), the pragmatic bioethicists believe that physicians need to attend to multiple considerations—not just the biomedical ones that are their traditional domain—when they make clinical decisions and recommendations. In an article titled "Bioethics and the Whole: Pluralism, Consensus, and the Transmutation of Bioethical Methods into Gold," Patricia Martin (1999) argued that bioethicists need to integrate a complex set of scientific data and diverse human values in order to transform ethical quandaries in medicine into consensual decisions. Achieving consensus for difficult medical decisions—such as the choice not to use heroic measures to treat an individual with a terminal condition—depends on paying careful attention to the biomedical facts of the matter as well as to a plurality of ethical values, including those of the patient, the patient's family and significant others, the members of the treatment team, the institution in which the patient receives care, and relevant legal statutes in the jurisdiction in which the care is delivered. There is no single set of clinical considerations or ethical theories to guide the physician and the patient toward the most appropriate decision-making process in the context of clinical complexity, ambiguity, and uncertainty.

The emphasis on a plurality of scientific and humanistic considerations in medical decision making—the second *p*—leads naturally to an emphasis on the genuine participation of the patient (and family members when appropriate) in these decisions—the third *p*. Martin showed how the process of achieving consensus in clinical decision making involves the physician in a complex and dynamic interpersonal situation, where the authoritarian decision making process of medicine in years past has given way to a process that is truly collaborative and democratic. Participatory clinical care empowers the patient (and his or her family members) by involving them as equal partners in the process of deliberation and clinical decision making. This approach helps to avoid the ethical hazard of rigid or authoritarian medical paternalism and respects core bioethical values of patient autonomy, informed consent, and personal dignity. As ethicist Michelle Carter argued in "A Synthetic Approach to Bioethical Inquiry" (2000), a participatory process ensures a "pragmatic, humanistic, and contextualized approach" to medical treatment. This approach builds on the ideal of "shared decision making" between physicians and patients that has been advocated by medical ethicist Dan Brock (1991). Respectful dialogue and empathic engagement with patients are core elements of a pragmatic medical ethics. The democratization of the doctor-patient relationship has drawn growing attention from medical ethicists in recent years. In the article "Clinical Pragmatism: John Dewey and Clinical Ethics," Franklin Miller and his colleagues (1996, 44) wrote:

Democracy in the clinic means that clinicians should strive to facilitate positive participation by educating patients about their conditions, inviting conversation aimed at a shared process of setting goals, and deliberating about alternative approaches to treatment and care. Clinicians must share power with patients and family members by subordinating the technical aspects of medicine, over which they maintain control, to the ethical aspects of determining, through dialogue and negotiation, what is good for patients.

As to the fourth *p* (the provisional approach), pragmatically oriented clinicians and bioethicists have written about the importance of managing the unpredictable and open-ended nature of all clinical work. There is a growing movement in clinical medicine to reflect on the deeply flawed nature of medical sciences, to deliberate carefully on how to cope with medical uncertainty, and to openly acknowledge (and attempt to reverse) unfortunate medical errors if they do occur. In the article "Patient Autonomy and the Challenge of Clinical Uncertainty," Mark Parascandola, Jennifer Hawkins, and Marion Danis (2002) integrated the pragmatic principles of participatory treatment and provisional explanation. "In situations where there is substantial uncertainty," they wrote, "extra vigilance is required to ensure that patients are given the tools and information they need to participate in cooperative decision making about their care" (p. 245). In a paper titled "Clinical Pragmatism: A Method of Moral Problem Solving," Joseph Fins, Matthew Bacchetta, and Franklin Miller (1997) similarly argued that pragmatic clinicians strive along with their patients to tolerate ambiguity and uncertainty in complex clinical cases. In the book *Complications: A Surgeon's Notes on an Imperfect Science*, Atul Gawande (2002) observed that even highly technical surgery, which may be justified by empirical evidence in support of its efficacy, is often plagued by unpredictability, chance, and error. "Medicine's ground state is uncertainty," he wrote. "And wisdom—for both patients and doctors—is defined by how one copes with it" (p. 229).

Although clinical pragmatism has received growing attention in bioethics and general medicine, there is a paucity of scholarship that addresses its specific applications to psychiatric practice. One notable exception is the article "American Pragmatism and American Psychoanalysis" by psychoanalyst Arnold Goldberg (2002), who delineated the relevance of principles of philosophical pragmatism to contemporary psychoanalysis, where no single school of thought has achieved widespread acceptance and confusion about the relationships among many approaches abounds. In keeping with the principles of American pragmatism, Goldberg argued that psychoanalysis is an instrumental enterprise that should be driven primarily by results rather than theories; that favorable outcomes are more likely to result from the liberal use of diverse concepts than from "some final, unifying, overarching theory that puts it all together into a neat package" (p. 246); and that psychoanalysts ought to view theory as a tool for coping with complex clinical cases rather than as a reflection of objective certainty about human behavior. Goldberg's paper focuses on psychoanalysis but does not apply the principles of philosophical pragmatism to general psychiatry, where the tension between the scientific approach (such as use of psychotropic medications) and the humanistic approach (such as use of long-term dynamic psychotherapy) constitutes the field's most pressing conceptual disorder. In fact, no major work has used philosophical pragmatism and dialectical reasoning to transcend the science/humanism divide in general psychiatry.

The relative inattention to pragmatism in psychiatry is unfortunate given that implementation of the four *p*'s—the practical, pluralistic, participatory, and provisional approaches to psychiatric care—could help clinical psychiatry to work through its conceptual disorder and bridge the science/humanism divide. Each of these four elements of classical American pragmatism is of critical importance to psychiatric explanation and treatment in the twenty-first century. Therefore, in the remainder of this chapter, I apply these four principles of classical American pragmatism and contemporary pragmatic bioethics to clinical psychiatry. The intention here is not to delineate a conceptual template to serve as a rigid and overarching explanatory model for all cases, but instead to highlight some key (and frequently neglected) principles that can help to guide clinical formulation and treatment in psychiatry. These pragmatic principles can help psychiatrists work within the science/humanism dialectic and point toward a more widely applicable, results-oriented approach to explanation and treatment of mental suffering in the twenty-first century. If psychiatry can employ pragmatic and dialectical reasoning to heal itself conceptually, the patients it aims to serve would be more likely to achieve the desired healing of their personal, emotional, and social lives.

The first implication of philosophical pragmatism for psychiatry is that psychiatric explanations ought to be practical (the first *p*) and thus are valid only insofar as they promote beneficial real-world results for individuals who seek mental health care. Like the American pragmatists, clinical psychiatrists ought to regard their theories not as ends in themselves but rather as tools for dealing with the practical challenges they confront each day in the clinic. By adopting a pragmatic position, of course, psychiatrists do not necessarily commit themselves to a particular viewpoint on the underlying structure of the universe. Consilience, in which all scientific knowledge is incorporated into a unitary system of understanding, need not be the ultimate goal of clinical observation or research in psychiatry. But that should not be taken to imply that psychiatrists should flout the legitimate findings of empirical science that may be relevant to diagnosis and treatment. Rejection of Wilson's consilience paradigm does not necessarily imply acceptance of Rorty's neopragmatism or of any postmodern view of psychiatric reasoning.

Psychiatric explanations are coherent and plausible insofar as they are effective in the course of clinical care and are subjected to continual questioning, testing, and reassessment. Although psychiatrists need not accept the reductive elements of Wilson's consilience paradigm, neither should they assume an antiscientific stance or repudiate the possibility of understanding and treating patients more effectively by employing the findings of empirical science.

The second *p* of American pragmatism is pluralism, which in psychiatry can be viewed as the notion that it is ethically and scientifically disadvantageous for psychiatrists to limit themselves to one side of the science/humanism dialectic in clinical work. In "The One and the Many," James argued that pragmatic thinkers aim to consolidate knowledge but also to acknowledge the reality of "a world imperfectly unified still, and perhaps always to remain so" (p. 79). Havens (1973), who introduced the term *pluralism* to modern psychiatry, applied this pragmatic idea by advocating a coherent, scientific approach to psychiatry but also pointing out the need to retain a multiplicity of clinically useful explanatory models, including the objective-descriptive, psychoanalytic, existential, and interpersonal models. Psychiatrists Paul McHugh and Phillip Slavney (1998), in *The Perspectives of Psychiatry*, similarly pointed to the need for multiple approaches to patient care, ranging from the biomedical "disease" approach to the psychological "life story" approach. The field is still struggling to implement methodological pluralism in meaningful ways. Unyielding fixation on a single, reductive theory of mental disorder can shortchange patients—such as Rafael Osheroff when treated at Chestnut Lodge (see page 16)—by depriving them of comprehensive care tailored to their unique situations and needs. Clinical treatment settings are no place to pursue a "pure" science that aims to describe the functioning of the brain but ignores ethical and practical implications of that science. Psychiatrists cannot allow their theoretical commitments or preferences to prevent them from treating their patients in a way that is open to acknowledging novelty and surprise and to learning something from patients that may call their theoretical models into question.

People enter psychiatric treatment with an astonishing array of problems, backgrounds, and needs. They generally wish to be understood and treated as individual persons, not as disease entities reducible to diagnostic labels. They strive to cope with and adapt to their situations in creative ways. Their difficulties are frequently long-standing and complex, and often result from a confluence of numerous constitutional vulnerabilities and psychosocial stress; this idea is often referred to as the "stress-diathesis model" of psychiatric disorder. Evidence has emerged to suggest that many mental disorders are caused or exacerbated by a panoply of neurobiological and psychosocial factors acting in concert. So it is no surprise that evidence has mounted to reveal that these disorders are best treated in a multimodal fashion, using a full complement of psychopharmacological and psychotherapeutic strategies. In addition, there is mounting evidence that the popular methods of complementary and alternative medicine can help to reduce stress, anxiety, and depression. Psychiatrist David Servan-Schreiber (2004) has described the efficacy of such approaches as acupuncture, physical exercise, and natural remedies like omega-3 fatty acids. Any ethically justifiable explanatory model for clinical psychiatry must recognize the pluralistic nature of mental suffering and the wide variety of approaches, both conventional and unconventional, that are available for treating it.

A psychiatrist's main commitment, therefore, should not be development of reductive theories of behavior per se—whether those theories are biological or psychological. But neither should the primary allegiance be to eclecticism or postmodernism or any other philosophy of complexity and disorder. While treatment settings often are not conducive to rigid application of empirical science, neither are they a place for postmodern rejection or devaluation of knowledge that has already been acquired, regardless of how incomplete that knowledge may remain. Even in the absence of a fully developed science of human suffering, psychiatrists should not succumb to the antiscientific temptation to reject the notion that they can acquire plausible and useful knowledge about human experience and behavior. Empirical science is helpful (and even indispensable) in psychiatric care, but mental disorders are complex and treating them usually occurs in the face of significant uncertainty. When empirical science provides sound evidence for the efficacy of a treatment, clinical ethics demands that the evidence be heeded. But in cases where there is less certainty (or no relevant empirical evidence at all), clinical decision making should not be wedded to any particular theory at the expense of concrete, practical considerations.

Instead, clinical psychiatrists' most abiding commitment ought to be to the individualized and specific needs of the patients they are treating. Drawing on James's notion of a pluralistic universe, they must have multiple explanatory tools available at all times. Meanwhile, drawing on the strengths of the empirical sciences, they must choose their diagnostic and therapeutic models carefully, with serious consideration of any available scientific evidence and expert consensus. To ensure good patient care, clinicians need to have many explanatory concepts at their disposal, but they should then use sound clinical judgment to refine their diagnoses and treatments in a practical direction. Clinical judgment, of course, is very difficult to define, but its core elements would include evidence-based hypothesis formation, consideration of a wide range of diagnostic possibilities, careful observation of a broad spectrum of clinical phenomena, flexibility to revise a clinical formulation on the basis of new evidence, and open-mindedness to consultation with other colleagues in situations that are characterized by complexity, confusion, and uncertainty.

This pluralistic approach would assist psychiatrists in the quest to achieve a conceptual synthesis between the extreme poles of explanatory consilience and disorder. By engaging in a dialectical process that aims to balance science and humanism in clinical interactions, the psychiatrist works along with the patient to construct a treatment plan that respects individual variation and complexity, but also makes judicious use of scientific reasoning. This dialectical pluralism entails a constant and steadfast commitment on the part of the psychiatrist to achieve the optimal balance of scientific and humanistic sensibilities, concepts, and methods for the sake of achieving the desired clinical outcome. The process of dialectical pluralism lends contemporary psychiatric meaning to the idea of methodological pluralism delineated by Peirce, James, Dewey, and other thinkers in the tradition of philosophical pragmatism. And it gives life to McCauley's co-evolution$_p$ in the current philosophy of science, which embraces the pluralistic idea that numerous approaches to scientific inquiry ought to reinforce one another in a never-ending dialectic.

Dialectical pluralism differs from other recent conceptions of psychiatric pluralism, such as the one espoused by psychiatrist S. Nassir Ghaemi in his book *The Concepts of Psychiatry: A Pluralistic Approach to the Mind and Mental Illness* (2003). Ghaemi's notion of pluralism is that there may be many relevant schools of psychiatric practice, but that only one approach will be appropriate in any particular situation. In limited cases (such as in clinical research studies of medications for a single psychiatric diagnosis), Ghaemi is correct that application of the concepts and methods of one school of psychiatric thought is appropriate in the clinical encounter. But unlike highly controlled clinical research, most real-world cases in general psychiatric practice are so complex—and most areas of psychiatric science are so poorly developed—that it is implausible to restrict the clinical formulation and treatment plan to just one conceptual approach. Unlike Ghaemi's notion of "pluralism," which tends to limit the psychiatrist to just one approach (even if a combination of approaches would have practical benefits), his notion of "integrationism" empowers the psychiatrist to draw on a broad range of conceptual approaches at any given moment in order to develop an effective clinical explanation and treatment. Ghaemi's integrationism is similar to my own notion of dialectical pluralism: both empower the psychiatrist in every clinical encounter to make use of relevant clinical science, to draw on and integrate several models as needed, and to cope with the bewildering complexity of most patients' clinical presentations.

Development of a clinical explanation occurs as a longitudinal process in which the psychiatrist, the patient, and others (such as family members or other clinicians working with the patient) collaborate and deliberate about the complex and dynamic aspects of any given clinical situation. This consideration leads to a third pragmatic principle that is central to contemporary psychiatric practice: full participation of the patient (and, when appropriate, other important people in the patient's life) in treatment planning. The American pragmatists rejected the notion that a single individual acting alone could acquire valid knowledge and instead suggested that truth is the outcome of a deliberative, social process that aims at identifying what works best in any given situation. Thus, rather than trying to force the patient onto a general and static explanatory template, the pragmatic psychiatrist works along with the patient as a partner in a longitudinal process of exchanging data and ideas about how best to proceed. While the clinician may be able to offer technical expertise on various aspects of human behavior, the patient also must participate as fully as possible to ensure comprehensive assessment and treatment. This interactive and deliberative process allows for the emergence of a genuinely participatory approach to psychiatric care. Some patients may need to be involuntarily hospitalized to ensure their safety or that of others, but even these patients still can participate in deciding how they will be treated, especially once they are stabilized. They may wish to sign an advance directive that will state how they wish to be treated when they are psychotic or otherwise unable to participate in clinical decision making in the future (Swanson et al. 2000).

When clinical formulations develop in the dialectical space between the poles of scientific order and humanistic complexity, employ a deliberative and collaborative approach, and aim to promote healthy functioning in the patient's best interest, McCauley's co-evolution$_p$ model—in which pluralistic approaches to scientific inquiry evolve together dialectically—becomes a genuine possibility for psychiatry. Such a model would draw on all the respective strengths of science and humanism, but temper them both with practical, ethical, and patient-centered considerations. It would embrace a pluralistic set of explanatory concepts and reflect "that cooperative tendency toward consensus" that Dewey, in "Experience and Nature" (1925), considered a hallmark of any pragmatically based empirical science. It would empower psychiatry to become a truly pragmatic activity that aims to integrate empirical science and ethical values in order to enhance the lives of people suffering with complex and multifaceted conditions, none of which we can fully explain or cure at this point in time.

This idea leads to the fourth pragmatic principle central to explanatory models in current psychiatry: the provisional nature of psychiatric explanation, which is consistent with the American pragmatists' notion of "fallibilism." As clinical psychiatrists acknowledge the elementary state of current understanding of human experience and behavior, they must remain open to novel approaches and formulate their cases in a rigorous and evidence-based fashion to whatever degree possible, but at the same time avoid taking the sometimes tempting leap of faith to presuming that current concepts are adequate or final. Considering that many formulations and treatments in psychiatry have proven ineffective in the past (recall, for example, the Osheroff/Chestnut Lodge case), it would be prudent for clinical psychiatrists to be curious about (and receptive to) more clinical complexity than currently can be conceived. In simple terms, psychiatrists should be humble about what they think and how they convey it to their patients. In an article titled "Education for Uncertainty," psychiatrist John C. Whitehorn (1963) warned that technologically oriented medical training can place physicians at risk of assuming "a pose of certainty" and "a phony attitude of omniscience" that compromise their capacity to relate to patients effectively and to consider alternative ideas that may be clinically useful. Some may argue the value of attaining certainty. But when clinical formulations are provisional and open-ended, psychiatrists can use scientific and humanistic approaches in a practical manner while also remaining open to novel approaches that may emerge in the course of further learning and reflection, fresh clinical experiences, or new and unforeseen research findings.

This trend may be seen at work in other sciences as well. The idea of provisional explanation is, in fact, a general principle of most contemporary scientific work. In an essay on the implications of the human genome project, philosopher of biology Richard Lewontin (2001) wrote that identification of the complete sequence of the human genome did not teach us very much about what it means to be human. An estimated 30,000 human genes, Lewontin noted, seem inadequate to explain the complexity and sophistication of human life—especially given that the mustard weed has as many as 26,000 genes. The search for biological complexity that mirrors the complexity of human life and behavior, Lewontin explained, has moved from the genome to the proteome, which is the set of all proteins produced by the human body. Elucidation of the nature of all proteins in the human body may lead ultimately to some significant advances in our scientific knowledge and our clinical capabilities. But considering the complexity of the human body and the failure of the human genome project to tell us everything we need to know about ourselves, one can reasonably suspect that the elucidation of the proteome would not constitute the final word on human biological functioning either.

Like modern biology, modern physics is increasingly well attuned to the complexities and indeterminacies of nature. In an article titled "Can Science Explain Everything? Anything?" physicist Steven Weinberg (2001) argued that even in the most basic science of physics, there will always be limitations on the certainty of explanations. Quantum mechanics, the foundation of modern physics, is rooted in uncertainty and indeterminacy. Rejecting the classical Newtonian view that the world is composed of physical objects whose interactions can be measured and predicted from an objective vantage point (in which the human observer is outside the field of study), contemporary quantum physicists believe that the physical world does not exist independently of human activity, that it can be understood only in terms of our interaction with it, and that it is changed by any attempt we make to measure and manipulate it (the Heisenberg uncertainty principle). They believe that physical events can only be predicted in terms of probabilities rather than certainties. The assumptions and findings of quantum physics reveal the indeterminacies of the natural world and of human behavior (which, of course, is part of the natural world) to be one and the same thing. As psychiatrists Bandy Lee and Bruce Wexler described in the article "Physics and the Quandaries of Contemporary Psychiatry: Review and Research" (1999), physics and psychiatry have converged on each other by way of their common interest in complexity and uncertainty.

As we have seen, explanatory completeness eludes us not just in the medical sciences but in the natural sciences as well. Humility and tentativeness are especially warranted in psychiatry, where all clinical formulations and treatment plans should be developed in a longitudinal and malleable fashion. Tolerating (and perhaps benefiting from) ambiguity in the clinical presentation is indispensable for sound patient care. For example, even if there is neurological pathology with explanatory and therapeutic relevance to a patient's condition, the clinician may profit from identifying other neurological, psychopharmacological, psychodynamic, or interpersonal factors affecting the patient's lived experience. Similarly, even if an individual was a victim of sexual abuse, the psychiatrist must investigate how the individual interpreted and coped with the trauma. There may be no identifiable causal bedrock, such as a brain lesion or psychological trauma, from which a mental disorder stems directly. Along these lines, philosopher and psychoanalyst Jonathan Lear (2000, 21) wrote that often "there is no Archimedean point, no explanatory end-of-the-line in a brute appeal to reality." Diagnostic assessments and treatment plans ought to acknowledge that clinical explanations are not determinate and fixed but open-ended and corrigible. Clinical care should be guided by available empirical science applied in a compassionate and patient-centered fashion, which hopefully will lead to pragmatic diagnosis and treatment without closing the possibility of incorporating previously unidentified factors.

Notwithstanding the trend toward provisional explanation in science, biological and psychological reductionists continue to presume that it is possible to achieve completeness and finality in explanations of human behavior. They believe that a fundamental goal of psychiatrists and neuroscientists ought to be the development of a single and complete explanatory model. This approach might appear to be tenable in cases in which the psychiatrist performs a cross-sectional, diagnostic evaluation of a patient at a specified moment in time. In such cases, the clinician may hypothesize that a patient's symptoms resulted from an identifiable intrapsychic conflict, an emotionally traumatic event, a neurological lesion, or an interpersonal conflict. This cross-sectional formulation might in turn prompt some important decisions about the short-term treatment intervention and the long-term prognosis. However, because human beings do not exist in isolated time frames but instead emerge from the past and project themselves into the future, the cross-sectional and reductive approach to case formulation in psychiatry has limited utility. Since human behavior is complex and multifaceted and ever changing, reductive clinical explanations in psychiatry often prove misleading and oversimplified.

This consideration does not imply that we must adopt a hopeless or postmodern sensibility about psychiatric science. Although reductive explanations are not well suited to evolving and uncertain circumstances and patient-care needs, clinical psychiatrists need not retreat into an unfocused, disordered eclecticism. Plausible and testable hypotheses, which emerge from the clinician's scientific knowledge base and experience of the patient at hand, are justifiable and useful if the clinician keeps in mind the relative indeterminacy of human behavior. The pragmatic approach in psychiatry can utilize the strengths, and minimize the short-comings, of both reductive science and eclectic open-mindedness. It heeds the empirical evidence but it avoids the reductive tendencies of conventional science by recognizing the practical, pluralistic, participatory, and provisional features of clinical explanation. At the same time, it starts from a commonsensical presumption that human behavior is complex and determined by a plurality of factors, but goes well beyond straightforward common sense by firmly rooting itself in any available empirical evidence and in the ongoing, rigorous testing of its claims.

Integrating science and humanism is the major challenge facing clinical psychiatrists today, a challenge that involves acknowledging the complexity of mental suffering but striving for scientific rigor. Twenty-first-century psychiatrists ought to pursue sound empirical science without falling into reductionism, but acknowledge individual variation and complexity without falling into eclecticism or a philosophy of disorder. A co-evolution$_p$ approach can help psychiatrists work through the evolving dialectic of science and humanism. The subscript p serves as a reminder of the *practical*, results-oriented nature of psychiatric explanatory constructs and therapeutic models. It indicates the *pluralistic* nature of diagnostic and therapeutic concepts that are needed in many clinical situations, as well as the *participatory* and collaborative nature of mental health care. It reminds clinicians of the *provisional* state of formulations and treatments in a science as incomplete as psychiatry. The four p's can guide the psychiatrist's hypothesis-driven, open-ended, multidimensional, and dialectical interaction with the patient in the context of an empathic, longitudinal therapeutic relationship. If their approach is practical, pluralistic, participatory, and provisional, psychiatrists in the twenty-first century will be in a favorable position to provide the scientifically and ethically sound care that patients desire and deserve. Chapter 3 contains clinical vignettes that will help to bring these ideas to life.

3

Pragmatism in Action: Clinical Cases

How might philosophical pragmatism be applied in the case of a particular patient? Consider the current possibilities when a patient seeks psychiatric care. The diagnostic and treatment approach that will determine the patient's care depends in large measure on the explanatory model of the clinician seen. If the patient sees an internist or clinical psychopharmacologist, he or she will likely receive psychotropic medication, the use of which will hopefully be supported by empirical evidence for its safety and efficacy. The patient may also be referred for some additional treatment, such as evidence-based CBT. But if the patient sees a psychodynamic therapist or a psychoanalyst, the recommendation for treatment might deemphasize the evidence-based approaches and the use of medications or standardized psychotherapies. The clinician in this case would take an idiographic approach that focuses on elucidating the patient's unique emotional experiences and psychological dynamics. Neither a scientific model nor a humanistic model is necessarily right or wrong in any given case, but it is clear that either one—if applied inflexibly or dogmatically—would run the risk of neglecting potentially relevant factors in the patient's treatment.

If, however, the patient ends up in the office of a psychiatrist who works in the pragmatic model I have delineated, he or she will meet a clinician who (1) focuses on achieving a practical outcome rather than working in strict accordance with a particular theoretical presumption; (2) assumes a pluralistic stance by considering both the scientific evidence and the patient's unique existential, psychological, and interpersonal situation; (3) invites the patient and, when appropriate, other key people in his or her life to participate intimately in all decisions about the nature of the treatment; and (4) acknowledges the provisional and open-ended nature of these decisions in the context of a longitudinal treatment. This pragmatic model may entail a creative combination of psychotherapy and psychopharmacology, which is increasingly recognized by both psychotherapists and psychopharmacologists as more effective in many situations than either approach alone. The pragmatic psychiatrist will make use of every applicable explanatory concept along the biopsychosocial continuum in order to collaborate with patients toward the goal of achieving integrative and beneficial treatment outcomes. This pursuit will heed and incorporate any scientific evidence that may apply to the clinical situation at hand, but will do so in a flexible, interactive, and humanistic fashion. It can and ought to be done without falling into the trap of postmodernism's lack of theoretical and practical clarity.

Because integration of science and humanism in psychiatry is a pragmatic process that is aimed at making a real-world difference in the lives of patients, it would help to supplement the theoretical arguments presented so far with some clinical case histories. The impoverished nature of strictly scientific or humanistic explanatory approaches in psychiatry—and the need to integrate the approaches in most clinical formulations—can be illustrated by consideration of the following clinical vignettes, in which a practical, pluralistic, participatory, and provisional approach helped to generate a results-oriented, patient-centered treatment plan. The patients described here, whom I have treated over the past several years, have been deeply disguised to ensure their anonymity.

Case 1

Laura first called me for an appointment because she recently had moved to New England and needed a prescription written for her antidepressant medication. In our initial telephone conversation to set up a time to meet, I sensed that she saw the appointment as an inconvenience and a necessary evil that she would have to endure in order to get the medication she considered so indispensable to keep her functioning in her part-time job and in her master's program in the social sciences. When she came to my office the following week, she told me a few facts about herself and reiterated her simple wish that I write her a prescription renewal for her antidepressant. Laura was dressed in black, had a pierced upper lip and tongue, and struck me as emotionally guarded. During the first few minutes of the meeting, I found myself wondering what kind of pain she had endured in her life that had led her to erect barriers to letting someone get to know her in even the most superficial way. After she related a brief synopsis of the 7-year history of her symptoms of depression, I told Laura that I would be happy to write her the prescription but that we still had about 40 minutes scheduled to discuss whatever was on her mind. She appeared skeptical and reluctant about speaking further, but said she would do so if I wished.

Laura told me that she was 22 years old and recently had graduated from a college in the Midwest, near where she had grown up. She lived alone in a studio apartment in a nearby city and had only a few friends and casual acquaintances in the area. She hoped to attend law school someday in order to become a public advocate, but she feared that she was not intellectually or emotionally capable of following through on this aspiration. She denigrated her academic and athletic achievements in high school and college, and she expressed disdain for herself over the fact that she was planning to begin a volunteer job in a legal aid clinic because she thought it would enhance her law school application in case she decided to pursue that possibility in the future. Laura's existence had become increasingly hollow, lonely, and bleak over the previous few years. She was convinced that antidepressant medication had preserved her ability to function day to day and to appear reasonably content to people with whom she interacted regularly at work and at school. But inside she felt as though she was emotionally decaying without anyone, including her closest family members, noticing that anything had gone wrong in her life.

Should I just write the requested prescription and send Laura on her way, back to her functional but gloomy everyday existence? Or was there some way I could reach her and form a connection that might allow her to share more of her suffering with me and possibly obtain some relief from how awful it had become? As I elicited more of Laura's history, I learned that she had a brother who lived in another state, but she was not close to him. In fact, she described her parents, brother, and others in her life in two-dimensional terms, as though they were cardboard figures rather than vital human beings. Toward the end of the session, when we had already moved past the scant discussion of her family life, she looked out the window of my ground-floor office, noticed it was snowing, and offhandedly mentioned that her sister Debbie had been a great skier. Her sister Debbie? I worried for a few moments that I had not been paying attention to Laura's story and had missed an important piece of information about a member of her nuclear family. But in fact Laura had neglected to mention Debbie up to that point. These kinds of gaps and oversights in patients' stories often mean nothing much, but sometimes they serve to cover over unconscious anxiety or even terror about confronting scary or painful feelings.

When I asked Laura to tell me more about her sister, she said matter-of-factly that Debbie had died 7 years earlier. I noted to myself that this 7-year time period coincided with the time Laura had been depressed and on antidepressant medication. After expressing surprise that she had lost her sister at the age of 15 and pointing out to Laura that she conveyed the information about her sister rather stoically, Laura replied that Debbie had committed suicide after a long battle with depression and self-destructive impulses. Debbie was 22 years old at the time of her suicide—exactly the same age Laura was now. After Debbie's death, the family discarded most of her belongings and put the rest of them, as well as any photographs of her, into boxes that remained out of sight in the basement of the family's home to that day. My initial hunch that Laura might need more than a prescription renewal now intensified into a conviction that bottled-up feelings—such as sadness, rage, and guilt around Debbie's death—were contributing to Laura's depression and despair. I wanted to make myself available to her for psychotherapy but knew realistically that she probably would not accept my help at that point. I said, "This year you are going to outlive your sister," and I noted that Laura was trying to hold back tears in response. I went on to say I would be happy to hear from her again if she wished to talk more about the troubling feelings this might raise. Laura replied that she would be fine with the medication prescription but thanked me for the offer of talk therapy. As she left, I found myself hoping to see her again before she would need another written prescription months later.

About 6 weeks after that initial consultation, Laura called to say that she had hit "rock bottom" and wanted to come to my office to talk things over. From there, we began a year-long psychotherapy process in which Laura struggled to articulate her thoughts and feelings about Debbie's death and her deep sense of aloneness in managing her emotions. Laura described her parents as good people who had always encouraged her to succeed in sports and school, and supported her financially as she considered the option of applying to law school. They had been devastated by Debbie's death to the point that they were completely unable to discuss Laura's emotions or their own in the aftermath of the suicide. The topic remained off limits in family conversations throughout the years that followed. Laura came to believe that these emotions were too overwhelming to be dealt with directly and that the loss of a family member to suicide was something to feel ashamed about. In the course of our discussions in psychotherapy, she gradually became more comfortable with the idea of talking about her feelings openly and came to learn that they did not have to be accompanied by shame or fear.

As Laura pursued this process over the next several months, she began to consider the idea of sharing more of her story with some friends from college and with a man at work whom she hoped to date. Her medication dose remained the same throughout this time, and it was the psychotherapy that seemed to give her hope that she could overcome her loneliness and despair. Compelling evidence that the process was working began to emerge. One year into the treatment, Laura reported a dream in which her parents had died and she hoped to be adopted. A number of people were in competition to adopt her but she was resistant to all of them because she could sense that they had their own selfish agendas. Suddenly she was sitting in a chair face to face with a man also seated in a chair, and she decided immediately that she wanted him to adopt her. They moved their chairs closer to each other and embraced, and at that point Laura experienced a sense of emotional excitement and intimacy that was entirely new to her. In our discussion of this rich dream, Laura and I agreed that she had experienced her parents as emotionally unavailable (and so in the dream depicted them as dead), that she wished to be cared for by someone who would help her understand her emotions, and that she needed to know that the person who was to "adopt" her did not have a selfish "agenda." We also agreed that the man who appeared at the end of the dream was me, sitting in my office chair across from her and trying to connect with her emotionally. While she acknowledged that she wished to be embraced and cared for by me, she also realized that the therapy experience had awakened in her a whole new set of loving feelings that she could bring to bear in her personal life.

Laura's case illustrates many of the core values of clinical pragmatism in present-day psychiatry. Evidence-based psychiatric science suggested that Laura had a significant family history of major depression that responded, albeit in a woefully inadequate way, to psychotropic medication. The scientific approach to her case, which supported the use of antidepressant medication, was helpful but clearly not enough. Dialectical pluralism suggested the need to introduce a more humanistic approach to understanding and treating Laura as well. The pluralistic approach allowed for the ongoing use of medication but also a deepening of the treatment experience with psychotherapy built on trust and an emotionally driven interchange between the therapist and the patient. The participatory-care aspect of Laura's treatment involved suggesting early on that psychotherapy may help her, but giving her space to decide on her own if and when to pursue it. A provisional approach to Laura's treatment was also critical. To assess the merits of Laura's multidimensional treatment, it would be important to see months and years down the line whether these hypotheses about her psychological dynamics really helped her to lead a fuller emotional life and to develop a richer set of relationships with others. As her therapy proceeds, clinical pragmatism requires that Laura and I continue to deliberate together about what approach in the sessions makes most sense for her in light of the practical challenges she faces in her everyday life.

Case 2

Michelle is a 30-year-old former actor whom I had the rare opportunity to treat in two separate contexts: first in the setting of a clinical research trial for an antianxiety medication, then in a long-term psychotherapy. She never had treatment for a long-standing pattern of anxiety, tension, irritability, gastrointestinal distress, insomnia, and intermittent panic attacks in which she would hyperventilate and sweat profusely. After reading an advertisement for a free psychiatric evaluation followed by treatment with either antianxiety medication or placebo, she decided that she had suffered with her symptoms long enough and that she finally needed to take action to improve her everyday existence. She was planning to get married in the coming year and wanted to feel like less of a "wreck" for the sake of her husband and their marriage. She understood that she had a 50 percent chance of receiving a placebo and that neither she nor the clinical researchers would know whether she received the drug or a placebo during the study (this was a double-blind study). She reasoned that if she could improve within the 6-week time frame of the study for no fee, she might not need to pursue an expensive course of outpatient psychiatric treatment, which was not covered by her insurance plan.

During the 6 weeks in the study, Michelle's clinical improvement was remarkable. By the second week, she felt less tense and keyed up at work, she slept well at night, her gastrointestinal discomfort diminished, and she suffered no further panic attacks. She complained of mild sedation and dizziness during the day, which may have been side effects of the study drug—though this remained unclear because of the double-blind nature of the study. Overall, she was very pleased with how she was feeling but was understandably confused about why she felt so differently as compared to how she felt before entering the study. This raised questions in our minds that arise in many psychiatric treatments, whether the setting is clinical research or general office practice: was the clinical change due to biological intervention (psychotropic medication) or was there something about the hope instilled in her by seeing an attentive physician each week to talk about the most private and troubling issues in her life? While we knew that we could not achieve certainty at the end of the research study as to whether she had responded to medication or had experienced a robust placebo effect, Michelle and I suspected it was the former, because dizziness and sedation are such common side effects of the study drug.

Despite the remarkable diminution of her anxiety symptoms within a week or two of the study, Michelle remained deeply troubled and dissatisfied with her lot in life. As the study progressed, she wished to use the sessions not to discuss somatic symptoms and medication questions, but instead to describe long-standing concerns about her tendency to inhibit herself emotionally in relationships and in a variety of situations in her life. She told me that she had abandoned her acting career in her midtwenties because she was unable to experience or express strong emotions when on stage. Her natural talent as an actor had allowed her to achieve success in a well-regarded college drama program and in some small parts in off-Broadway plays in her early twenties. But her anxieties and inhibitions prevented her from reaching her potential and eventually rendered it impossible for her to pursue drama as a viable career path at all.

Michelle described a parallel set of concerns about her sexuality and her relationship with her fiancé. When they first dated during senior year in college, she recalled experiencing an ardent passion for him, enjoying their active sexual relationship, and achieving powerful orgasms on a regular basis. Over the past several years, however, these feelings had waned to the point that they had not had sexual intercourse for 6 months at the time she entered the study. Her lack of strong feelings for her fiancé and her inability to express passion on stage or in the bedroom left Michelle feeling purposeless, discouraged, and worried about her future. Her sexless relationship and her new job as an administrative assistant for a financial services company were no outlets for the many passions that stirred inside her, but that she could not effectively access or express. As her symptoms of generalized anxiety resolved in the study, her frustration about the absence of excitement, pleasure, and passion in her life intensified. She deeply missed the high-pitched feelings she remembered from better days when she was still acting and was energized by her sexuality.

These feelings persisted at the end of the research study and so Michelle decided to do weekly psychotherapy with me despite the fact that her insurance company would not assist her financially. Acting on the presumption that she had received the study drug rather than the placebo, she went onto a prescribed antianxiety medication at the conclusion of the study. In psychotherapy over the next several weeks, she continued to vent her frustrations with the absence of passion in her daily life. At one point during a session in the third month of therapy, I asked her if she could recall times in her childhood when she felt strongly about something but ended up suppressing these feelings. She immediately "flashed" to a memory that she had never shared with anyone and that she herself had not thought about for many years. At the age of 5, Michelle recounted, she had been masturbating in her bedroom and enjoying this recently discovered activity. Suddenly, her father entered the bedroom unannounced and saw what she was doing. He had a look of horror on his face and told her sternly to get up and never do what she was doing again; he made no attempt to minimize her shame or to discuss anything about sexuality in a way a 5-year-old child could grasp. Michelle said that she could still evoke the feeling of utter humiliation that this experience had induced in her.

Michelle felt slightly embarrassed to report this story to me in therapy but she felt extremely relieved to share it and to acquire some understanding about the origins of her tendency to experience strong passion, yet to suppress that passion or shut it down completely. Although this new understanding did not immediately change the nature of her relationship with her fiancé, it did allow her to feel less distraught about the situation and more hopeful that she could work it out. She had come to recognize that the problem was not her future husband's inability to sustain her emotional or erotic interest, but her own susceptibility to inhibiting her passions because of a deep-seated fear of their power and the shame that could be associated with their expression. Uncertainty remained about whether Michelle's traumatic memory of being discovered masturbating by her father was a basically accurate reflection of reality, an exaggerated version of something similar that had occurred, or a fantasy she created that encapsulated her concerns about passionate sexuality (what Sigmund Freud referred to as a "screen memory"). Whatever the case may be, discussing this memory in therapy helped Michelle to feel that her inhibitions were intelligible, manageable, and amenable to change for the better.

Having identified a plausible source of her inhibitions, Michelle decided a couple of months later that she could no longer afford the weekly psychotherapy sessions but that she wished to continue taking antianxiety medication. She was beginning to note some modest improvement in her relationship with her fiancé and they restarted their sexual relationship, though its intensity was diminished and its frequency was irregular. She also began to consider more appealing job options that would allow her to make better use of her interpersonal skills. After 6 months of weekly therapy, we terminated the treatment with the understanding that it could restart if her symptoms recurred or progress in her relationship with her fiancé stalled.

Michelle left therapy feeling she had achieved important practical results despite the fact that our formulation of her anxieties and inhibitions was far from certain. Was her primary problem a biologically determined anxiety disorder that would require long-term treatment with psychotropic medication? Or was it an inhibited personality style that emerged from the traumatic childhood memory and would require long-term insight-oriented psychotherapy? Were the biological and psychological issues equally in play and could they best be conceptualized as standing in a complicated and endless dialectical relationship to one another? Would additional contributing factors come to light if Michelle continued in the psychotherapy or entered four-times-per-week psychoanalysis? The pragmatic approach to Michelle's case took a diversity of contributing factors—including her response to medication and to discussion of a painful memory—into account and used them flexibly to help her achieve some beneficial (albeit limited) results. In the end, the formulation of her troubles was provisional and necessarily left open more questions than it answered. As Michelle's married life and career unfold in the future, she may return for additional treatment that builds on this formulation or trades it in favor of new hypotheses more in keeping with a new set of challenges in her life.

Case 3

Another patient I saw in individual psychotherapy was Jay, who had suffered with melancholic depression for many years: his symptoms included depressed mood, hopelessness, absence of pleasure and enjoyment, and low motivation for work and socializing. A complex array of neuropsychiatric deficits likely contributed to his melancholia. For example, he had a remarkably strong family history of mood disorders, suggesting a genetic vulnerability. He likely had Asperger's syndrome, a pervasive developmental disorder with neurological underpinnings, in which the affected individual is quirky and odd, has trouble understanding social cues, and tends to focus on the trees rather than on the forest. In addition, Jay responded quite well, with significant relief of his melancholic symptoms, to antidepressant medications with strong effect on the neurotransmitter dopamine, but not to some other medications with more robust effect on the neurotransmitter serotonin. This clinical observation suggested that perhaps his depressive syndrome was caused in part by a dopamine deficiency in his brain.

The scientific formulation and treatment of his melancholia had been beneficial but inadequate. When his treatment with me began, he reported that he had tried several antidepressant medications but only a very brief psychotherapy. The medications had helped him feel much better, though he continued to feel sad, numb, empty, and isolated from others. In his depressed state, he remained obsessively focused for many years on an idiosyncratic pornography habit. He had accumulated a large collection of "paper dolls" assembled from mainstream and pornographic magazines, and he spent hours pursuing this activity. He would find photographs of clothed, attractive women in magazines and cut out the pages; then he would find photographs in pornographic magazines of women who had a similar skin tone and other features, his goal being to "cut and paste" the pictures so that the face of the clothed woman could be combined with the body of the nude woman, resulting in a composite photograph that he found stimulating. He organized and archived these pictures in files in his so-called hobby room at home.

Jay seemed to focus on fragmented parts of women's bodies and had difficulty regarding them as three-dimensional people. A tendency to focus on parts rather than wholes is fairly typical of individuals with Asperger's syndrome, so Jay's pattern of focusing on fragmented parts of women's bodies could be understood as a manifestation of his developmental disorder. After all, explaining and treating Jay's illness reductively—as a disorder of brain functioning—had been fruitful insofar as it led to treatment with certain medications that helped him achieve partial relief of his melancholia. But no combination of medications had been successful in relieving all of his symptoms: he remained chronically dissatisfied with his life and derived little enjoyment from things that used to give him some pleasure, such as reading. Together we decided, therefore, to pursue a weekly psychotherapy in which we would examine the psychological dynamics and meanings of his condition, with the goal of discovering whether a humanistic approach would complement the scientific approach and yield more favorable practical results in his everyday life.

Jay and I agreed that he would continue on his medication but also meet for weekly therapy sessions in addition. Within a few sessions, he began talking about blows to his self-esteem that he had suffered years earlier, many of which involved his feeling extremely humiliated either by his mother or by women in whom he had developed some romantic interest. For example, he recalled his mother's repeatedly confusing his name with that of his father, as though they were "interchangeable, generic male family members"; this had left him feeling "invisible." This idea of interchangeable people seemed to relate to the nature of his pornographic activities, which involved fragmentation of women whom he did not regard as real, whole human beings. In the course of psychotherapy, he achieved the insight that perhaps in his pornography activities he liked to see women fragmented and placed in embarrassing and compromised positions because women throughout his own life (beginning with his mother) had so often humiliated him.

Over the course of months, Jay displayed a far wider range of emotion when discussing his depression, pornography, and lack of social relationships. He seemed less detached in therapy as time went on and he became more affectively engaged in the sessions. Most notably, five months into the therapy he stopped using pornography entirely and said that his melancholic symptoms had abated. Rather than spend hours with pornography, he developed new friendships and began a consulting business in his professional field. He also showed signs of becoming more interested in the subjective experiences of other people around him. All of this occurred with no change in his medications or, in fact, any other clear biological change. The cause of the diminution of Jay's melancholia and the shame associated with his pornographic habit, of course, is complex and may never be fully knowable. Based on changes that accompanied a psychotherapeutic exploration of the meanings associated with his pornographic obsession, however, it seems plausible that psychological and interpersonal factors had contributed importantly to the development (and the resolution) of his symptoms.

At the same time, Jay clearly had a biological susceptibility to that very set of symptoms. The plurality of scientific and humanistic factors that surround Jay's condition could tempt the clinical psychiatrist to simplify matters and adopt a reductive approach to his case that focuses on medication management alone. The opposing temptation would be to see the wide range of biological, psychological, and interpersonal considerations in his case as disconnected and utterly confused. Considering that plausible (yet tentative) hypotheses about his condition were available, it would be unwarranted to slip into either a reductive materialism or a slapdash eclecticism. Pragmatic principles applied in the case of Jay guided the explanation and treatment of his condition to a pluralistic and collaborative approach in which the clinician and the patient together developed plausible, evidence-based, and testable hypotheses.

Psychotherapy gave Jay and me an opportunity to understand his complex symptoms in a coherent but open-ended fashion. A dialectical understanding of his depression and troubling pornography habit emerged as we came to recognize the dual contributions of his biological disorder and the long-standing deficits in self-esteem that dated back to his interactions with his mother and other women. When we focused in on his biological disorder, we could put the origins of his troubles in perspective and we found a more effective medication regimen, but we also found ourselves pulled back to thinking about the deficits in self-esteem that underlay his unhappiness. Conversely, when we delved into his humiliating experiences with his mother and other woman in his life, he at times felt angry and overstimulated; at such times, considering the role of his neurodevelopmental disorder and medication regimen diffused this emotional intensity but allowed us still to deal with important aspects of his treatment. Understanding the dialectical interplay between scientific and humanistic factors in his life seemed to empower Jay to replace a pornography obsession with the more fruitful endeavors toward which he began to direct his attention, such as his consulting business and his social life. The practical goals we had defined at the outset of his therapy had largely been achieved. Nonetheless, as some symptoms resolved, others issues (such as his rage at people who had hurt him) began to emerge and opened up new chapters in his ongoing therapy and the provisional understanding of his struggles.

A misstep that I made in the second year of Jay's treatment became a focal point of his pragmatically oriented therapy and an important learning opportunity for both of us. With Jay's permission, I published an account of our work together in a professional journal in which I disguised his identity, focused on certain aspects of his emotional suffering, and provided a highly exaggerated account of his somewhat formal interpersonal style (Brendel et al., 2002). After the article was published, I presented Jay with a copy of it with the caveat that I overemphasized some aspects of his case but had played down others in order to make certain didactic points. Despite this warning, Jay felt hurt and enraged by some elements of my written portrayal, such as my use of the terms *stilted*, *pedantic*, and *blind* to certain social cues, such as those that signify the end of a therapy session. Feeling guilty about upsetting Jay in this way but also intrigued by the clinical and ethical issues this experience raised, I presented the situation to a medical school ethics consortium and wrote up an account of the specific course of events and the general issues they highlighted (Brendel 2003a). This follow-up article was published side by side with an essay written under a pseudonym by Jay on what he had experienced in reading my write-up in a journal article (Carter 2003), as well as commentaries by several clinicians with an interest in the ethics of writing about patients (Halpern 2003; Howe 2003; Joffe 2003; Mitchell and Truog 2003).

The follow-up publication provided a unique opportunity for me to reflect on my preconceptions and missteps, and for Jay to gain a voice about his own treatment experience in an article in the professional medical literature. In terms of clinical pragmatism, the follow-up publication was a participatory experience in which Jay and I collaborated on trying to understand a thorny situation and to transform it into a learning experience with good practical results for Jay. As Jay saw me grapple with the guilt and shame I experienced as a result of upsetting him, he began to feel that I finally understood how much guilt and shame he had suffered in his own life for so many years. It was possible that my own struggles with this situation allowed me to empathize more effectively with Jay's sense of shame and humiliation, and for Jay to feel more understood by me than he had before. As we explored these issues over the ensuing months, I was impressed and moved by Jay's openness to expressing powerful feelings and by his willingness to give the ongoing therapy process a chance to transform such a deeply troubling experience into an opportunity for personal growth and clinical change. The pragmatic approach to Jay's case entailed a creative, coconstructed, patient-centered, and therapeutic response to a complex and disquieting clinical situation that had resulted in large measure from my own oversights, blind spots, and missteps in the second year of an otherwise unproblematic therapy.

Case 4

Adam is a 25-year-old homosexual white man who is completely blind and has many neuropsychiatric problems (including seizures, bipolar disorder, and attention deficit disorder) as well as a complex personality disorder, for which he is treated with a combination of psychotherapy and medications. Adam was born prematurely, weighing just 28 ounces. He was treated with toxic levels of oxygen in an incubator, which resulted in severe damage to his retinas and permanent blindness. He had a history of inattention, forgetfulness, hyperactivity, and behavioral problems dating back to childhood, but he was not diagnosed with attention deficit disorder until age 22, at which time he was started on a medication for that disorder (methylphenidate) by his primary care doctor. Extensive neuropsychological testing at age 24 indicated that he had remarkable strengths in the verbal sphere (conversational fluency and reasoning abilities) but less proficiency in performance tasks, such as reading in Braille. Because of his blindness, seizures, inattention, and mood instability, he required a great deal of external structure and support in order to function well in everyday life.

He was not suicidal when I first met him, but 6 years earlier, at age 19, he had taken a potentially lethal overdose with suicidal intent and had been admitted to an intensive care unit. He had started valproate—a medication for both seizures and bipolar mood swings—at age 18. Some of his seizures involved left-sided numbness and tingling followed by convulsions, loss of consciousness, and urinary incontinence; others were marked by speech arrest and inability to move parts of his body but a normal awareness of his surroundings. Once he started taking valproate, he experienced fewer seizures and also less frequent and intense mood swings. However, he continued to have intermittent episodes of mania and depression, which often occurred when he neglected to take his medication. The manic episodes were characterized by euphoric mood, grandiose ideas, insomnia, pressured speech, reckless spending, and sexual indiscretions (such as unprotected sex in bars with strangers). The episodes of depression were marked by sad mood, loss of interest in other people, and a sense of hopelessness and worthlessness.

Adam's father was alcoholic and his mother had frequent mood swings. The childhood home environment was chaotic and confusing. For about a decade, starting when Adam was 4 years old, his mother had a male lover who also lived in the home. On countless occasions, Adam was present in the bedroom as his mother and her lover had sexual intercourse; they seemed to assume he would not notice because he was blind. His parents divorced when he was 14 years old, and his grandmother sued for (and won) custody of him. Adam experienced the court battle between his mother and his grandmother as extremely traumatic. At age 19, Adam was emotionally devastated by the untimely death of his father. At age 21, he moved to another region of the country to be with a male lover and to receive vocational training. From there he was referred to a school for the blind in New England, where he lived on campus and attended classes for a few months. He soon met his roommate and lover, spent most of his time off campus with him, and left the school shortly thereafter.

Adam described two episodes in which he had been sexually molested as a child, the first at age 8 by a teenage male schoolmate and the second at age 12 by an older male cousin. Adam initiated consensual sexual activity with men at age 16 and had never been involved in a sexual relationship with a woman. He tended to date men who were several decades older than he was and were willing to play both paternal and sexual roles. For example, in his early twenties Adam became romantically involved with a 67-year-old man, who provided him with emotional support when Adam informed his family that he was gay and as a result felt like an "outcast." During that same time, he lived with another male lover, also in his midsixties; Adam left that relationship because he felt that that man verbally abused him.

Shortly before I began treating him, he had been admitted to a psychiatric hospital because of irritability, insomnia, hypersexuality, and paranoia (i.e., fear that his lover and roommate, who is 40 years his senior, was trying to poison him). While hospitalized, Adam expressed the grandiose delusion that he had come back to life to complete "the mission of Billie Holiday." Admission to the hospital was preceded by friction between Adam and his lover stemming from Adam's sexual involvement with another man, who was also four decades older than Adam.

When I met Adam, he had just left the psychiatric hospital because his mood was more stable, but his treatment remained as scattered and disorganized as Adam himself. Numerous physicians remained involved in his care and he requested that they prescribe him methylphenidate because he was convinced that it had helped him to lose weight, to pay attention, and to elevate his mood; they refused to do so because of the risk that it would precipitate mania or seizures. In fact, Adam continued to have seizures and an electroencephalogram (EEG), a test that measures the brain's electrical activity, revealed several independent sources of seizures on both sides of his brain. His neurologist suggested that Adam's seizure disorder continue to be treated with valproate and the gradual addition of lamotrigine, another medication that helps to prevent seizures and bipolar mood swings.

Adam had a few appointments with a psychotherapist but did not feel engaged in the therapy process. The goal of his referral to me was to connect Adam with a new clinician with whom he might form a meaningful attachment and who could combine the medication management and the psychotherapy. Adam soon began coming to weekly appointments on a regular basis. He was driven to the clinic and guided up the stairs each week by his live-in lover, a steady and reliable figure who was gentle with Adam, provided him financial assistance, and helped him organize his medications at home. At the same time, though, Adam continued a romantic relationship with another man, a destabilizing force who provided passionate sex but encouraged him to drink alcohol and not take his prescribed medications.

During our initial sessions, Adam continued to ask for prescriptions for methylphenidate and persistently made the same request of the numerous other physicians who had treated him in the past. After much discussion over the next few weeks, however, Adam and I—in consultation with his other physicians—reached an agreement that only I would prescribe his psychoactive medications. He agreed to take prescribed medications only and to stop taking methylphenidate when I assured him that his concerns about weight gain, attention deficits, and depression would be vigorously addressed by other means. Within 2 months, he had come off methylphenidate and was being treated effectively with valproate and lamotrigine only. He took the initiative to place himself on a high-protein, low-carbohydrate diet to control his weight and subsequently did not request more methylphenidate.

The relationship with his lover became platonic but he continued to live with him. However, he continued the relationship with the other man, but lamented that he was controlling and did not support Adam's desire to take his medications and to achieve more independence. Adam was no longer delusional about Billie Holiday at that point and, in fact, did not mention her name until 14 months into our work together, when he spoke in realistic terms of his strong identification with her. His relationship with his controlling lover reminded him of one of the singer's lyrics, which Adam remembered as "I ought to hate him yet I love him so. I'm born to be in love with a no-good man."

A crisis ensued when Adam's ex-lover (with whom he was still living) expressed frustration that they were no longer sleeping together and stated his desire that they move into separate apartments. At first, Adam could not imagine the prospect of living on his own and became extremely anxious. Over the next several months, however, he began to look forward to the independence that this move would afford him. Plans were made for him to move into his own apartment with homemaker services and other necessary social supports. Before preparations could be completed, unfortunately, Adam ended up living on his own when his roommate was admitted to the hospital for a medical illness. Adam became scared and paranoid at home and was not prepared to take care of the basic activities of daily living, such as cooking. He was briefly admitted to the psychiatric hospital for stabilization and started on a low dose of the antipsychotic medication olanzapine, which helped to diminish his anxiety and paranoia.

After Adam was discharged and the necessary support services were in place, he moved into his own apartment. He broke off the relationship with the controlling lover but maintained regular contact with his former lover and roommate, who had moved to a separate apartment in the same building and still brought him to therapy appointments. For a time while managing medications without assistance, Adam missed some doses of valproate and again had seizures. Once his friend assumed the responsibility of helping him with this, Adam took his valproate regularly and the seizures abated. He had sufficient stability at this point to think about a return to a vocational program. He began deeper exploration in psychotherapy of his conflicted relationships with his male lovers and their roots in traumatic early life experiences of emotional chaos, sexual abuse, and loss. Themes about dominance versus subservience in relationships became increasingly prominent as he strove to achieve greater independence and a stronger sense of personal autonomy and effectiveness.

As his treatment progressed, Adam expressed relief that one clinician was attending to multiple aspects of his psychiatric condition. Physicians throughout his life appropriately attributed his problems with mood instability, paranoia, and inattention to the biologically based seizures, bipolar disorder, and attention deficit disorder. What attracted less attention from both Adam and his clinicians was a clear pattern of unstable and inconsistent "object relations" (i.e., relations with important people in his life) that was rooted in his turbulent early childhood experiences of abuse and loss. This pattern manifested itself later in Adam's life in his chaotic, frustrating, and sometimes abusive relationships with older male lovers and father figures. The pattern also manifested itself in unsatisfying and inconsistent relationships with his physicians, some of whom ended up feeling exasperated by him and prescribing medications that could be detrimental to his condition. In short, Adam never really had the opportunity to feel safe with (and depend on) an older person—whether a family member or a lover or a clinician—whom he could regard as trustworthy, consistent, and committed above all else to Adam's best interest.

When Adam was given the opportunity to invest his trust in (and stake his well-being on) a therapeutic relationship with a dependable clinician who could address the biological and psychosocial dimensions of his existence, he stabilized his life, complied with a safe and effective medication regimen, remained free of seizures and psychosis, and oriented himself toward a future of more independent functioning and fulfilling relationships. The increased structure and organization of his treatment reflected the increased focus and resolve he began to develop in his everyday life. Trusting one primary clinician also emboldened him to seek a monogamous relationship in which he felt respected and believed his emotional needs could be satisfied. Feeling safe and cared for in a therapeutic relationship that attended to multiple biological and existential concerns, Adam also came to participate more actively in his own care. Within a year of beginning treatment, he had lost over 30 pounds by way of diet and exercise—and he no longer demanded methylphenidate or any other medication that could be harmful in light of his complex neuropsychiatric condition. In his weekly psychotherapy sessions, he became increasingly proactive in deciding on and exploring the issues he considered most salient. In the language of clinical pragmatism, he had become a true participant in his own treatment.

A core pragmatic lesson that can be drawn from the treatment of Adam is that psychiatrists and patients are served well by a dialectical process that enables them to use both scientific and humanistic concepts flexibly in order to fashion integrated clinical formulations and to implement effective, humane treatments. In Adam's case and others like it, clinical data that are gathered from neurological examinations, laboratory studies, EEGs, and neuroimaging studies need to be supplemented by consideration of factors such as the patient's object relations, capacity for adapting to stressful circumstances, long-standing personality traits, and social situation. Even when a biological disease causes abnormal behaviors (seizures, mood instability, and attention deficits in Adam's case), understanding the patient's condition usually calls for a pluralistic formulation that captures its complexity and empowers clinician and patient to develop an individually tailored treatment plan. Psychiatrists who favor multidimensional case formulation (Perry, Cooper, and Michels 1987, 546) have argued that "the presence of nondynamic factors—genetic, traumatic, organic, and so forth—does not preclude the value of understanding a patient's psychodynamics."

Understanding the patient's condition also calls for a provisional attitude and open-mindedness to the possibility that the formulation can evolve, or even change radically, in light of new circumstances or clinical data. In Adam's case, for example, it turned out that he actually benefited from methylphenidate when it was added to his medication regimen in the second year of treatment to help him concentrate more effectively on his new job selling Internet services from his home. When used in combination with valproate, lamotrigine, and a consistent psychotherapy relationship, methylphenidate did not provoke seizures or mania; on the contrary, it seemed to play a helpful role in the further stabilization of his mood and behavior. In our dialogue about whether to initiate methylphenidate, Adam felt that he had a new and powerful experience with another man: he said that my willingness to consider methylphenidate for him gave him hope that a man in his life could understand his needs and respond to those needs respectfully and thoughtfully. In the early part of our work together, Adam had transferred his long-standing distrust of men onto me as his therapist. But with reliable care over many months, Adam came to regard me as a benign and compassionate "object," which empowered him to believe that he could find a friend and a lover with these same character traits. In fact, by the third year of treatment he had established a healthy, loving, nonabusive, and monogamous relationship with another man.

In a published account of Adam's treatment (Brendel et al., 2001, 182), a discussant of the case—psychiatrist Jonathan Florman— addressed key pragmatic issues this case highlights, including the practical, pluralistic, and provisional dimensions of psychiatric reasoning and treatment:

This case illustrates the central truisms of clinical neuropsychiatry. First, we see how our quest for neuropsychiatric precision—with regard to etiology, prognosis, and treatment—is often elusive, thwarted by the multidimensional complexities of the patient. Second, a psychodynamic perspective always enriches our understanding of the neuropsychiatric patient; the neurodevelopmental framework is continually modified by early experience, in particular by the presence or absence of a safe, nurturing environment. We cannot know to what degree the outcome here might have been different, had Adam been more fortunate in his early life experience. Third, and perhaps most important, this case illustrates how thoughtful and consistent care from a team of providers can make a real difference for even our most complex and compromised patients. Finally, a word on Billie Holiday, a telling choice as the object of Adam's identification and fantasy. Her soulful voice, extolling the burdens of love and loneliness, sings an appropriate anthem for Adam. She embodies a blend of passion and pain—a life colored by abusive relationships and heroin addiction—that must seem familiar to Adam. Billie Holiday's self-destructive excesses brought her career, and her life, to an early end. Perhaps one goal of Adam's treatment should be to enable him to sing the blues without succumbing to them.

Cases 5 and 6

Mark and Lyle, both men in their midtwenties whom I treated in individual psychotherapy, had been living in New York City in 2001 when their lives were irrevocably changed by the September 11 terrorist attacks on the World Trade Center. Lyle was in his apartment across the street from the twin towers when the planes struck that morning, and he was trapped for the next several hours with no telephone links and intense fear that he would not escape from the building alive. Mark was at his office in midtown Manhattan when the planes struck. However, his wife Jenny, who usually went to work at 10:30, happened to go in early to her office on one of the high floors of the south tower that day after having spent time with Mark because she was worried about his upcoming surgery. Mark tragically lost his wife in the terrorist attack that morning; meanwhile, it would later turn out that Lyle would gain a wife in the aftermath of the turbulent events of September 11.

However, in the immediate weeks after the attacks, Lyle stopped going to work, burst into tears uncontrollably each day, and suffered with severe insomnia, anxiety, and agitation. By the end of September, he left New York and moved to New England (where he had graduated from school the previous year) to be with his girlfriend. But his symptoms continued and so he entered psychiatric treatment in mid-October, at which point he met diagnostic criteria for posttraumatic stress disorder (PTSD), with a host of symptoms that included nightmares, flashbacks, hypervigilance, avoidance of television coverage of the event, and fear of returning to New York to pick up his belongings. During the initial therapy session he noted severe hopelessness and a sense of dread, in addition to the acute posttraumatic symptoms. In accordance with widely accepted evidence for the optimal treatment of PTSD, an antianxiety medication was prescribed and provided some relief of the PTSD symptoms. In addition, Lyle agreed to meet in weekly psychotherapy for emotional support in the context of the abrupt and entirely unforeseen changes in his situation.

In the first few months after September 11, Mark fared much better than Lyle even in spite of Mark's unfathomable loss of the woman he married and with whom he had intended to start a family and buy a new home. In the immediate aftermath of the attacks, Mark took off a couple of weeks from his work at an advertising firm and he joined a support group for men in the New York City area who lost a spouse that day. He often cried and felt overcome with powerful and indescribable emotions, but was generally able to compose himself quickly and proceed with his day-to-day activities. In addition to attending the support group, he met with an individual counselor a few times, but felt that it added little to his mourning and recovery. He did not see a psychiatrist and took no medication for anxiety, sleep problems, or depression; he returned to full-time work by October.

Looked at from the standpoint of their overall functioning in mid-October, Lyle and Mark exhibited very different responses to the events of September 11. Although he did not lose anyone close to him that day, Lyle had feared for his life during the hours he was trapped in his building, and in short order he developed a wide range of symptoms that met diagnostic criteria for PTSD. Mark, on the other hand, was not in close physical proximity to the World Trade Center, but he lost the woman he had married and with whom he intended to spend the rest of his life; he grieved her loss but did not develop any severe posttraumatic symptoms. If Mark were to receive a formal psychiatric diagnosis at that point, it would have been a mild adjustment disorder or bereavement reaction.

Their responses up to that time, however, proved to be misleading when their lives were assessed several months after the original traumas. Lyle, for his part, formed a rapid and robust therapeutic alliance with me and in the course of two weeks, with a combination of antianxiety medication and psychotherapy, his PTSD symptoms resolved. Despite his initial reluctance to enter psychotherapy, he said that he had come to value the weekly sessions above everything else in his life at the time. Lyle clearly was skilled at forming a relationship and using it to power his emotional growth and to move his life forward. By Valentine's Day of 2002, he and his girlfriend were engaged to be married and were planning a large wedding. He felt guilty that the terrorist attacks of September 11, which caused so much suffering for so many people, actually led to his achieving a more balanced and fulfilling life. He managed this sense of guilt by talking about it openly in the therapy sessions and resolving to transform it into a greater appreciation of his own good fortune, redoubled efforts to cherish the people closest to him, and a decision to embark on a new career path that would allow him to contribute more meaningfully to others.

On the contrary, Mark's life began to deteriorate during the 6 months after September 11. Although he found some solace in his peer support group, he became increasingly withdrawn and lonely. He felt slighted by Jenny's parents, who did not include him in numerous decisions following her death, such as what to do with her personal belongings that were still in their home. In the spring of 2002, he was notified that parts of her body had been identified; this news led to disagreement with his wife's family as to whether the remains should be viewed and whether they should be cremated or buried (and, if buried, where that should be). Anger and resentment toward Jenny's family had been building in Mark for several months. In May, he resolved to leave New York City and move back to New England (where he had grown up) to live with his own parents. At that point he met diagnostic criteria for major depression on the basis of his sad mood, loss of previous interests, lack of energy and motivation, and thoughts about suicide. We began to meet and I suggested that he initiate treatment with antidepressant medication and psychotherapy.

Unlike Lyle, who seemed relieved and enlivened by the therapy sessions, Mark seemed guarded and reluctant to immerse himself in any kind of treatment. He reported that in high school and college he had been able to form superficial friendships, but did not maintain or deepen those friendships because he would come to find flaws and shortcomings in other people as he got to know them better. In sharp contrast to Lyle, he did not naturally and spontaneously form a meaningful psychotherapy relationship that could build a stronger sense of self, interpersonal connection, and hope for the future. These personality differences between Lyle and Mark were not apparent in a cross-sectional assessment of their states of mind and functioning during the initial weeks following September 11. But 6 months later, they turned out to be more predictive of Lyle's and Mark's respective mental states and overall conditions than were the earlier differences between them with respect to acute symptoms of PTSD.

In the initial weeks after the September 11 attacks, an intelligible account could be constructed as to why Mark had an expected grief reaction but did not suffer a marked posttraumatic stress response: he was far from the World Trade Center during the attacks, had warm memories of his wife, and knew that she had been trapped in the tower as a result of the love for him that had brought her into Manhattan to spend time with him early that morning. Similarly, a plausible account could be offered as to why Lyle's posttraumatic anxiety was so severe in the wake of the attacks: he had experienced a life-threatening trauma in a city where he had few friends and family members, and where he disliked his 80-hour-per-week job at a large investment bank. From a cross-sectional standpoint in the autumn of 2001, one might have rested satisfied with these clinical formulations. But a few months later, these formulations had been turned on their heads, as Lyle recovered and got engaged while Mark retreated into himself and became more symptomatic.

New and very different explanations of how Lyle and Mark got to this point in their lives became available in the spring of 2002, based on such factors as the capacity to form a meaningful relationship. In the long run, of course, these new accounts could be as misleading as the original accounts formulated in the autumn of 2001. Indeed, it is quite possible that, like Lyle, Mark could do very well over time. In fact, many considerations speak in Mark's favor, such as his emotional connection with his deceased wife and his persistent work with his support group. Thus, it would be as unwarranted to state that Mark's long-term prognosis is poor on the basis of his condition in the spring of 2002 as it was to state that his prognosis was favorable on the basis of his initial resilience in the autumn of 2001. Similarly, one must be cautious in assessing Lyle's prognosis. There is no reason to suspect future psychopathology in the absence of another life-threatening event, but one cannot yet say whether he will experience severe anxiety reactions on future anniversaries of the September 11 attacks or whether he will develop a long-term phobia of high-rise buildings, which he has tended to avoid since the attacks.

A reductive approach to these cases would suggest that Lyle's and Mark's patterns of behavior after September 11 ultimately could be explained on the basis of scientific findings, such as the demonstration of genetic differences in their vulnerabilities to anxiety and PTSD or of psychological differences in their capacities to cope with trauma and loss. An eclectic approach, on the other hand, would suggest that their reactions were determined in a hopelessly complicated way by such factors as their genetic makeups, inborn temperaments, personality traits, social situations, and experiences of horror and helplessness on September 11 and in the ensuing months. The reductive formulation would apply scientific theory to the clinical data but, by excluding the multiplicity of psychological and social factors that characterize their unique situations in life, would run the risk of oversimplifying Lyle's and Mark's complex, evolving neurophysiological and emotional reactions to their respective traumas. The eclectic formulation, on the other hand, would incorporate on an equal basis a whole host of factors spanning the biopsychosocial spectrum but, by failing to concentrate in particular on the most salient factors in each case, would run the risk of being unfocused and conceptually muddled. The reductive and the eclectic formulations both would the run the risk of sacrificing what works best in Mark's and Lyle's unique situations for what the respective explanatory models hold to be true from the standpoint of their theoretical commitments.

A pragmatic alternative to these reductive and eclectic formulations would involve developing scientifically plausible but tentative hypotheses that could be tested—and thus confirmed or refuted—continuously over time. In accordance with the pragmatic approach, these hypotheses would be tested for their practical benefits (or lack thereof), would be open to embracing a plurality of explanatory concepts, would seek the participation of the patient in these decisions, and would remain provisional and open-ended. For example, a partial explanation of Lyle's symptomatic improvement ought to be rooted in neurobiological principles, such as the likelihood that certain antianxiety medications (which he received) will be effective in treating the symptoms of post-traumatic stress. But in itself such an explanation of Lyle's progress over the course of 6 months following September 11 would be reductive and incomplete. A more comprehensive explanation of his personal growth and evolution should also include a pluralistic set of psychosocial principles, such as his ability to form a meaningful therapeutic relationship that enhances his life. Regardless of how advanced our understanding of the genetics and neurobiology of PTSD may be in the future, it would be unlikely that one could explain Lyle's existential changes on a scientific basis alone and avoid any consideration of what the psychotherapy relationship meant to him as a unique individual. Although it is possible that future scientific developments will allow psychiatrists to identify genetic traits that predispose people to particular patterns of interpersonal relatedness (such as introversion or extroversion), no scientific discovery of this sort could fully explain why a particular individual such as Lyle, at a particular moment in time, could or could not make use of an interpersonal relationship to move his life forward.

These antireductive considerations do not imply that an eclectic approach is the only or best option for clinical explanation in psychiatry. On the contrary, the pragmatic psychiatrist would remain open-minded to the notion that further discoveries in such areas as psychiatric genetics could help explain why a patient like Lyle reacted as he did to a traumatic experience. New drug development may also render the biological treatment of PTSD more effective in the future. The pragmatic psychiatrist's hypotheses would carefully consider relevant empirical research on psychological responses to terrorist attacks (e.g., Schlenger et al. 2002) and recommendations for appropriate treatment of PTSD as outlined in expert practice guidelines (e.g., Expert Consensus Panels for PTSD, 1999). Any assessment of Lyle's long-term prognosis should be formulated in a careful and rigorous manner that considers scientific evidence on the biological determinants of PTSD but remains tentative and open-ended. At the same time, any hypothesis about why Lyle improved as he did—and what his ongoing treatment should or should not entail—should include careful consideration of his inner world and personal situation, should be established with his active participation, and should remain amenable to revision in light of new information.

As it turned out, Lyle continued to explore his inner world in the context of psychotherapy, and in so doing he continued to feel that he made critical strides at a major turning point in his life. Within a few weeks, he found that he no longer needed antianxiety medication, as the focus of his everyday life and his therapy sessions changed from acute symptoms to his long-term career goals and his plan to get married the following year. In the course of treatment over several weeks, Mark's acute situation also stabilized and he decided to discontinue psychotherapy at that point. Although he found the prescribed medication helpful, he decided that talking about his troubling emotions at that point in time was overwhelming and counterproductive, though he left open the possibility that psychotherapy could be helpful to him in the future. The practical, pluralistic, participatory, and provisional approach to Mark's and Lyle's care helped to ensure that they received the kind of treatment they desired, that it made use of the limited but helpful evidence available to guide the treatment of PTSD, and that it integrated a broad spectrum of scientific and humanistic considerations that were relevant to understanding both their troubling symptoms and their individual personalities. The four *p*'s of clinical pragmatism in psychiatry helped to heal Lyle and Mark to the extent that they could be healed in light of the traumas they had experienced as a result of the September 11 attacks.

Discussion

The narratives of Laura, Michelle, Jay, Adam, Mark, and Lyle may be dramatic and unique, but they certainly are not atypical. In these cases, scientific reasoning played an important role in establishing relevant psychiatric diagnoses, suggesting possible neurological contributions to the psychiatric presentation, and guiding an appropriate use of laboratory studies and psychotropic medications. At the same time, scientific reasoning was insufficient to explain all aspects of the patients' subjective experience, meaningful actions, and patterns of interpersonal relations. Even as scientific reasoning helped to structure and to organize the treatment, attention to the humanistic complexity and uncertainty inherent in each case was equally helpful in individualizing the case formulation and treatment approach. The unending challenge of articulating the appropriate relations among a broad swath of scientific and humanistic approaches was the central challenge in these cases and, indeed, is the key challenge in most cases in clinical psychiatry today.

Clinical work with patients like Laura, Michelle, Jay, Adam, Mark, and Lyle will be enhanced if psychiatrists can employ scientific reasoning when it is helpful and avoid falling into the antiscientific traps of eclecticism or postmodernism. At the same time, psychiatrists need to remain open-minded to the complex meanings of people's behavior and to the possibility of changes in their patients that they could not have predicted. Dialectical pluralism embraces a broad range of explanatory concepts and recognizes the dynamic interplay among them, but it calls on the psychiatrist to integrate those concepts in a way that aims at concrete practical results, respects the patient's collaborative involvement in the therapeutic process, and remains mindful of the open-ended nature of case formulations and the need to revise the formulations in light of new circumstances. Applying the principles of clinical pragmatism and working with the dialectic of science and humanism can guide the twenty-first-century psychiatrist and patient toward the therapeutic goals that together they seek to define.

4

Pragmatism and the Mind/Body Problem

Just as clinical psychiatrists can enhance patient care by attending to the conceptual basis of their explanatory models, philosophers of mind can glean from psychiatric reasoning some important lessons about the roles of scientific and humanistic concepts in explaining human action. The debate between science and humanism can be addressed fruitfully in psychiatry by way of the four *p*'s of clinical pragmatism, which provide a conceptual and practical framework for addressing complex challenges in psychiatry. But pragmatism also deserves to be considered seriously in the related debates on the mind/body problem that rage among philosophers. The considerations in previous chapters suggest that extreme versions of scientific reasoning (such as Wilson's consilience) and of humanistic reasoning (such as postmodernism) are equally untenable in clinical psychiatry. Analogously, two such positions in the contemporary philosophy of mind—one that goes to a scientific extreme ("eliminative materialism") and one that goes to a humanistic extreme ("mysterianism")—are unsupportable on pragmatic grounds. Explanatory theories in philosophy of mind and clinical psychiatry are misguided if they veer toward either pure science or pure humanism. The core principles of philosophical pragmatism can rescue both psychiatry and philosophy of mind from the dangers that emerge at their ideological extremes.

One aspect of the tension between science and humanism is the mind/body problem, which is a critical concern in both philosophy of mind and clinical psychiatry. Unprecedented growth in neuroscience has prompted some theorists to hypothesize that psychological explanations are unscientific and will become obsolete as neuroscience advances. Other theorists have countered that, even in the face of a rapidly maturing neuroscience, psychological concepts remain relevant and necessary in many circumstances. Debates on whether every dimension of human thought and behavior might be explicable in purely physical terms pervade recent literature in the philosophy of mind. In a volume titled *The Mind-Body Problem: A Guide to the Current Debate*, philosophers Richard Warner and Tadeusz Szubka (1994, 13–14) wrote that the essential question philosophers nowadays pose about the mind/body problem is "whether the scientific program of a fully mind-independent description and explanation of nature extends without fundamental modification to the description and explanation of the mind." In other words, our growing capacity to describe brain functioning from the level of genes to the level of neural networks leads us to ask whether human experience and behavior are just as amenable to scientific analysis as is the physical world itself.

Mind/body issues in philosophy and psychiatry can be approached from two vantage points: the ontological and methodological. Considered first from the ontological standpoint, the mind/body problem addresses what kinds of things minds and bodies are. Is the mind identical to the brain or is it a nonphysical entity distinct from the brain? Most contemporary philosophers of mind and psychiatrists are ontological materialists who reject the notion that the mind can be understood as a nonphysical entity separate from the brain (an exception among thinkers in this area is John Eccles, a neurophysiologist with a philosophical bent, whose commitment to a nonmaterial mind or soul stems from religious concerns). Philosopher Jaegwon Kim (1996, 3), who like so many of his colleagues is an ontological materialist, wrote that the notion of a disembodied mind "has never gained a foothold in a serious scientific study of the mind and has also gradually disappeared from philosophical discussions of mentality." In light of growing scientific evidence that shows close connections between brain functioning and behavior, ontological materialism—the position that all entities, including the human mind, are physical—has become the only widely accepted position.

From a clinical standpoint, physicians' encounters with brain-disordered patients provide rich and compelling evidence for ontological materialism and an intimate relationship between altered brain functioning and disturbed cognition, affect, and behavior. Contemporary clinicians, for the most part, interpret their work with patients with well-defined brain pathology to exclude the possibility of a disembodied mind as postulated by such philosophers as René Descartes. For instance, in his book *Descartes' Error: Emotion, Reason, and the Human Brain*, behavioral neurologist Antonio Damasio (1994) argued against Descartes's notion of a disembodied mind by presenting clinical vignettes and research findings that demonstrate the direct links between brain pathology and disturbed emotions, thoughts, and behaviors. When a clinician can understand a patient's depression as a direct result of a stroke or a tumor in gray-matter regions of the brain's left frontal lobe, there seems no need to presume any nonphysical mental entity to account for the symptoms.

In addition, from a primarily theoretical standpoint, Kim (1996, 4) pointed out that there is a "near consensus" among contemporary philosophers of mind that postulating an ontologically distinct, nonphysical mind leads to "too many difficulties and paradoxes without compensating explanatory gains." Those who believe in a disembodied mind must presume a realm of physical things such as brains (Descartes's *res extensa*) and a second realm of things that are unobservable (*res cogitans*). In so doing they defy Occam's razor, the doctrine that urges us to presume the existence of only those entities that we require in order to understand and to get by in the world; on this account, ontological materialism is preferable to Descartes's mind/body dualism because it is more conceptually parsimonious. Besides violating Occam's razor, those who view mind and brain as ontologically distinct cannot account for how two completely different sorts of things—brains and minds—might interact. The ontological materialist's rejection of a disembodied mind seems to dissolve the intractable philosophical problem of accounting for how mental events and brain events could actually affect one another.

But ontological materialism has not abolished the mind/body problem. In spite of their rejection of disembodied, brain-independent mental events, most philosophers of mind and psychiatrists continue to employ both psychological and neuroscientific concepts in explanations of both ordinary and pathological human behaviors. This is the case because the mind/body problem also has an important methodological dimension. Considered in this fashion, the mind/body problem addresses whether objective, natural scientific concepts are adequate to explain all human behavior or whether in some cases it is appropriate or necessary to employ subjective, psychological concepts as well. In psychiatry, where ontological materialism is a widely accepted principle, a critical methodological concern is how it might become possible to integrate psychological and neurological clinical data so as to formulate sound explanations and treatments of mental disorders. Whereas the philosopher's goal is to achieve theoretical clarity on the nature of the mind/body relationship, the clinical psychiatrist's goal is to assess and treat people with mental illnesses. Although their goals and methodologies are distinct, clinical psychiatrists and philosophers of mind share a common mission to clarify what they mean when they talk about the mind, the brain, and the complicated relationship between the two.

In an essay titled "Can We Solve the Mind-Body Problem?," philosopher Colin McGinn (1994) argued that this problem is intelligible but completely insoluble because it is impossible to grasp the property of the brain that underlies consciousness. While McGinn is a scientific realist who acknowledges that there must be a "property of the brain that accounts naturalistically for consciousness," he also believes that fundamental limitations on human thought processes render us "cognitively closed with respect to that property" (p. 102). Philosopher of mind David Chalmers (1996), in his book *The Conscious Mind: In Search of a Fundamental Theory*, took this position a step further by arguing that conscious experience can only be understood outside a materialist framework and that there is, in fact, no property of the brain that could ever account for human subjectivity. Philosopher of mind Thomas Nagel (1974) similarly argued in favor of respecting the inherent gap between observable brain functioning and unobservable subjective experience in his famous essay "What Is It Like to Be a Bat?," in which he argued that understanding the scientific basis of the bat's sonar system provides interesting information about the bat's neurophysiology, but tells us nothing about what the bat actually experiences subjectively. Applying this theory to human beings, neuroscience may be able to tell psychiatrists a great deal about how people's brains function, but it can never tell them anything about what it is like to be the patient from the standpoint of the patient's lived experience.

These philosophical stances on the mind/body problem have been called "mysterianism" because of the mysterious nature of the property of the brain that causes consciousness (McGinn's theory) or the mysterious nature of conscious experience itself and the impossibility of saying anything meaningful about it in the language of neuroscience (Chalmers's and Nagel's theories). The strength of these ideas lies in their humility about the complex relationship between mind and brain, and their openness to many methods for understanding various dimensions of human life.

But how do these theories apply to clinical psychiatry? A problem with mysterianism lies in its reluctance to entertain the plausibility of scientific and philosophical advances in this area. It may be unnecessarily pessimistic to be resigned to the futility of conceptualizing the mind/body relationship, and it may be premature to foreclose the possibility of constructing plausible and testable hypotheses regarding this relationship in the future. Psychiatrists who adopt mysterianism as the basis of understanding the mind/body relationship in clinical work may develop a defeatist attitude when it comes to attempting to apply emerging psychiatric science to their work with their individual patients. At the very least, mysterianism provides psychiatrists with no conceptual foundation on which to think about the causal connections between biological therapies (such as psychotropic medications) and patients' subjective responses to such therapies.

Then again, other theories go to the opposite extreme of mysterianism, overestimating the role and the promise of reductive science. Wilson's theory of consilience and the unity of explanation is a prominent contemporary example of such scientific overzealousness. Like Wilson, some philosophers of mind suggest that if human beings are physical creatures without disembodied minds, their experience and behavior ultimately should be explained with physical concepts only. They believe, in other words, that accepting ontological materialism necessarily requires adopting methodological materialism. This idea has been advocated by contemporary philosophers of mind such as Paul Churchland (1981, 67), who has characterized "folk psychology"—the ordinary psychology that people use to understand one another in the course of everyday life—as "a theory so fundamentally defective that both the principles and the ontology of that theory will eventually be displaced by completed neuroscience."

Churchland (1981) argued that psychological concepts are particularly unhelpful for explaining "the nature and dynamics of mental illness." In fact, he recognized that mental illness caused by identified brain dysfunction provides the strongest argument in favor of eliminative materialism. "So long as one sticks to normal brains," he wrote (1988, 46), "the poverty of folk psychology is perhaps not strikingly evident." He went on to say, however, that the poverty of psychological explanation, and the rationale for eliminative materialism, become abundantly clear "as soon as one examines the many perplexing behavioral and cognitive deficits suffered by people with damaged brains" (p. 46). Considering that ordinary "folk psychology" remains imperfect after being employed for many centuries and that neuroscience has begun to elucidate the causes of some human behaviors (such as the abnormal behaviors of individuals with known brain dysfunction), Churchland (1981, 75) suggested that psychology is now "a serious candidate for outright elimination."

Churchland's theory poses significant challenges for philosophers and psychiatrists because there is some historical precedent for elimination of entire modes of scientific explanation on the basis of empirical discoveries that reveal the invalidity of the earlier explanatory models, such as Ptolemaic astronomy and alchemy. When scientists demonstrated that presuming the existence of oxygen could help them better understand and manipulate the natural world, the earlier concept of phlogiston was not just revised or fine-tuned—it was eliminated from scientific reasoning entirely and replaced by the concept of oxygen. In the realm of human behavior, there was a time in Western history when people explained each other's actions by invoking divine forces (such as the Furies or a deus ex machina), but divine explanatory tools have been excluded from modern scientific vocabulary as behavioral scientists have found ways to predict and explain human action from the standpoint of empirical study. Scientific findings have revealed that some clinical disorders can be explained and treated biologically, and the recent history of psychiatry has suggested a clear trajectory away from psychological and toward neurobiological explanations. Does this fact imply that the latter is in the process of eliminating the former?

Unprecedented neuroscientific advances throughout the twentieth century gave psychiatrists increasing hope that disorders that had appeared psychogenic would yield to biological explanations. For instance, clinical changes associated with late-stage syphilis, such as personality changes, were widely thought to stem from the afflicted individual's moral character until the twentieth century, when it was discovered that these behavioral changes actually resulted from the infection of the central nervous system by the microorganism *Treponema pallidum* (Quetel 1990). The new understanding of neurosyphilis as an infectious disease was supported by empirical findings that it could be treated effectively with malaria fever therapy and later with penicillin and newer antibiotics (Braslow 1995). Similarly, before the neuroscientist Lewy discovered in 1914 that paralysis agitans (Parkinson's disease) resulted from pathological changes in the brain's basal ganglia, the illness was viewed primarily as a psychosocial disturbance (Roth and Kroll 1986). Today, it is well accepted that Parkinson's disease results from the degeneration of dopamine neurons that project from the brain stem's substantia nigra to the basal ganglia and control the planning and initiation of complex motor acts (Kopin 1993). What's more, some types of major depression that frequently affect patients with Parkinson's disease are explicable in terms of deficiencies in levels of the neurotransmitters serotonin and dopamine in critical brain areas (Sano et al. 1990; Taylor and Saint-Cyr 1990).

Analogously, whereas psychoanalyst Silvano Arieti (1972) had described catatonic schizophrenia—a devastating form of schizophrenia in which the patient can become mute and unable to move—as "predominantly a disorder of the will," clinical psychiatrists today explain most cases of catatonia in neurophysiological terms. Recent neuropsychiatric research has suggested that catatonia can best be understood as a crippling motor disorder that is associated with mood disorders and schizophrenia but also with a whole range of neurological disorders, such as epilepsy, toxic exposures, and brain damage (Rogers 1991; Carroll et al. 1994). Obsessive-compulsive disorder (OCD), which is characterized by intrusive and repetitive thoughts and actions that the affected individual cannot control, is yet another syndrome clinicians have attempted to explain in neuroscientific vocabulary, as a disorder of a network of key neurons in the brain. Two experts on OCD noted that "with the advent of new imaging techniques and the discovery of novel drug treatments, OCD is no longer considered to be a psychological disorder" (Robertson and Yakely 1996, 839).

Contemporary psychiatrists often favor neurological over psychological vocabulary when explaining abnormal thoughts and behaviors of people with identified brain disease. That is, they often assume that brain pathology signifies what philosopher Michel Foucault (1965) called a "fall into determinism." For example, when a patient with frontal lobe disease develops a behavioral disorder, the initial tendency is to explain the symptoms in terms of the deranged neuronal pathways. A case in point is Damasio's (1994) evocative description of his patient Elliot, a dependable husband and businessman who exhibited a major personality deterioration after he developed a benign but large brain tumor (a meningioma) that compressed both frontal lobes of his brain. Even having suffered substantial frontal lobe damage from the tumor and the surgery to remove it, Damasio noted, Elliot remained physically and intellectually intact. But Damasio went on to say that the root cause of the distressing change in Elliot's personality and judgment was damage to his frontal lobe and that as a consequence of this damage "his free will had been compromised." Because the meningioma can be understood as a fall into determinism, neurological concepts appropriately took priority in the case formulation.

Such clinical realities must render us skeptics about the validity of current mental vocabulary, since we can foresee that in years to come the disorders we currently explain in psychological terms may become explicable in neurological terms as our scientific knowledge and clinical acumen improve. Since many clinical disorders that at one time were considered psychogenic have been successfully reconceived in neuroscientific terms, it is natural that contemporary psychiatrists would want to entertain the fundamental tenets of eliminative materialism in the setting of identified brain disease. "In confronting the entire range of psychological dysfunctions," Churchland (1995, 183) wrote, "we have done far better by looking for structural failures or abnormalities in the brain, for functional failures in its physiology, for chemical abnormalities in its metabolism, for genetic failures in its original blueprint, and for developmental hitches in its maturation." Eliminative materialism, Churchland's theory, extends beyond the domain of abnormal behavior associated with brain dysfunction, however; the theory holds that all human action will one day be explained biologically. This goes for normal behavior of healthy people as much as for deranged behavior of people with brain disorders. Churchland (1981, 75) thus looked forward to a day when psychological concepts could be eliminated in toto and replaced by the concepts of "particle physics, atomic and molecular theory, organic chemistry, evolutionary theory, biology, physiology, and materialistic neuroscience."

The critical question Churchland raises is whether ontological materialists are justified in formulating explanations of human behavior that employ concepts from disciplines other than the physical sciences, such as psychology. If we are biological creatures whose minds are ontologically inseparable from our brains, is there ever a legitimate place in explanations of people's behavior for conceptual tools provided by psychology, such as beliefs, desires, wishes, and fantasies? If we are going to accept the principles of ontological materialism and construe the contemporary mind/body problem as a distinctly methodological challenge, it becomes important to identify what role the concepts of psychology might have in explaining the behavior of complex biological creatures like ourselves. As philosopher Charles Taylor (1985, 186) wrote, the challenge is to decide whether it is feasible to develop "a non-dualistic conception of man which is nevertheless not linked with a reductivist notion of the sciences of man." Can the contemporary philosopher and psychiatrist function as both an ontological materialist and a methodological pluralist? Philosophical pragmatism not only empowers them to adopt such a hybrid stance, but actually requires them to do so when confronting ethical challenges such as the provision of appropriate patient care. Dogmatically applying philosophical approaches like mysterianism or eliminative materialism to the practice of clinical psychiatry would be imprudent and potentially harmful to patients.

But what philosophical position on the mind/body relation can serve as a suitable alternative? The goal here is to identify a conceptual model that respects philosophers' and psychiatrists' widespread belief in the principles of ontological materialism but at the same time allows for pluralistic explanations of people's behavior, explanations that draw on a broad range of psychosocial concepts in addition to the concepts of neuroscience. When applied in the clinical setting, this model would have to be focused on helping patients achieve their practical goals and considering whatever empirical evidence applies to the situation at hand. In the current philosophy of mind, the best approach to support these pragmatic values is "nonreductive materialism," which holds that no disembodied human mind exists (ontological materialism) but that understanding people's experience and behavior requires a vast array of conceptual tools (methodological pluralism). In a book chapter titled "Nonreductive Materialism and the Explanatory Autonomy of Psychology," philosopher Terence Horgan (1993) delineated the foundations of this philosophical model and the importance of its practical applicability. Horgan noted that a multitude of explanatory concepts ("microphysical, neurobiological, macrobiological, and psychological") are available to account for human activity and experience, and that the concepts we employ at any particular time ought to be driven by our practical needs rather than by theoretical presumptions. "Typically, certain context-relative features of discourse," Horgan wrote, "will determine, in a given situation of inquiry, which sort of explanation is most appropriate for the purposes at hand" (p. 298).

Nonreductive materialism in the philosophy of mind is consistent with McCauley's co-evolution$_p$ approach in the philosophy of science. Like Horgan, McCauley (1996) argued that philosophers ought to be "pragmatically minded," and that this means in part that they should aspire to reason scientifically even as they work with a pluralistic set of explanatory tools to solve particular theoretical and practical problems. There are numerous forms of nonreductive materialism in contemporary philosophy, but they all share a fundamental belief that ontological materialism and methodological pluralism are compatible. The theory of "emergent properties," for example, holds that complex physical systems like the human brain have characteristics and functions that can only be accounted for by using a diversity of languages, including the language of psychology (Bunge 1977; Karlsson and Kamppinen 1995). The theory of "multiple realizability" suggests that mental states can be realized in an infinite number of brain states, that mental concepts refer to a different set of phenomena than neurological concepts, and therefore that mental concepts cannot be eliminated from scientific discourse. In this vein, philosopher Donald Davidson, who articulated the theory of "anomalous monism" (1980), argued that a particular mental event is identical to a distinct brain event, but that general types of mental events (such as joy, pain, or depression) lack a delimited set of corresponding brain events. Because there is no fixed relationship between a general type of mental event and a specifiable brain event, neurological discourse is inadequate to fully describe human life and mental vocabulary is irreducible to physical vocabulary.

The pragmatically oriented philosopher and psychiatrist recognize that ontological materialism does not require that we discard pluralistic explanations, because the ontology of human life and the methodology to treat people clinically are separable. Clinical pragmatism empowers the psychiatrist to regard patients as physical beings, but to use a broad array of physical and nonphysical concepts to understand, explain, and treat them in clinical settings. Pragmatic arguments against extreme theories in the philosophy of mind (including mysterianism and eliminative materialism) are necessary for overcoming the mind/body problem, especially in a clinical context. A pragmatic rebuttal to eliminative materialism can be synthesized out of the novel cross-disciplinary arguments of the Nobel Prize–winning psychiatrist/neuroscientist Eric Kandel and the psychoanalyst Susan Vaughan, who recognize a practical need for dynamic psychotherapy in the treatment of many patients, but also point to research suggesting that its efficacy may derive from the observable alterations it induces in the brain. They adhere to ontological materialism by recognizing that psychotherapy changes the patient's brain functioning, while they adhere to methodological pluralism by advocating the need for clinical care that attends to the complex biological, psychological, and interpersonal matrix in which patients live.

Whereas Churchland (1995, 183) doubted psychiatrists could "fix a genuinely broken brain just by talking to it," Vaughan presents scientific evidence that they do just that all the time. Characterizing herself as a "microsurgeon of the mind," Vaughan (1997, 3) depicted psychotherapists and psychoanalysts as agents who help the patient alter his or her brain by way of talking and listening. She invoked the famous neuroscientific experiments conducted by Kandel on the sea slug *Aplysia*, which revealed that gene expression and testable nerve cell functions can be changed by the sea slug's experiences in its environment and its remarkable capacity to learn and adapt to change. Kandel (1979) offered an analogy between how the sea slug's neurons respond to environmental stimuli and how those of a person's brain change in psychotherapy: "It is only insofar as our words produce changes in each other's brains that psychotherapeutic intervention produces changes in patients' minds" (p. 1037). Likewise, Vaughan (1997), in a chapter of her book creatively titled "The Sea Slug on the Couch," suggested that psychotherapy can induce "specific alterations in neuronal and synaptic functioning such as those that occur in *Aplysia*" (p. 67–68). The long time course required for real psychotherapeutic changes may be due to the fact that alterations in gene expression and neuronal functioning only take place over prolonged periods of time. From the pragmatic standpoint, it is conceivable that neuroscience will not eliminate psychology: on the contrary, neuroscience actually seems to be lending psychotherapy further empirical support. Psychotherapy can be understood as a pragmatic endeavor that benefits patients while rooting itself in brain science and ontological materialism.

While there are substantial differences between the nervous systems of a sea slug and a human being, Vaughan's notion is plausible. Besides Kandel's work on *Aplysia*, experimental work with human subjects has suggested the feasibility of altering human brain physiology with psychotherapy alone. In one set of studies, cognitive-behavioral therapy (CBT) was employed as a treatment and its efficacy was assessed by neuroimaging techniques that revealed how brain physiology changed as a result of the therapeutic intervention. The researchers (Baxter et al. 1992) evaluated treatment responses over a 10-week period of eighteen OCD patients: nine subjects only received CBT and the other nine only received treatment with the medication fluoxetine (Prozac). In both groups, the investigators discovered that the patients who had a favorable clinical response (i.e., significant decrease in their OCD symptoms) also had clear evidence on functional scans of their brains, conducted at the beginning and the end of the research trial, of decreased glucose metabolism in the right caudate nucleus of the basal ganglia, an important brain structure considered to be a key part of the neuronal network that is disturbed in OCD patients.

Further studies are needed to evaluate whether long-term psychodynamic psychotherapy and psychoanalysis effect changes in relevant brain areas, as the Baxter studies have shown that short-term CBT can do for individuals with OCD. If such findings could indeed be replicated, they would help to confirm Kandel's hypothesis that scientists may be able to understand the neurological mechanisms associated with psychotherapeutic change. In his article "A New Intellectual Framework for Psychiatry," Kandel (1998, 460) looked ahead to a future where neuroscience may become another tool that helps to explain, confirm, and validate the practical efficacy of psychotherapy:

Insofar as psychotherapy or counseling is effective and produces long-term changes in behavior, it presumably does so through learning, by producing changes in gene expression that alter the strength of synaptic connections and structural changes that alter the anatomical pattern of interconnections between nerve cells of the brain. As the resolution of brain imaging increases, it should eventually permit quantitative evaluation of the outcome of psychotherapy.

Such neuroscientific findings clearly would not lead to the elimination of psychological approaches or psychotherapy but perhaps, for distinctly pragmatic reasons, to their more widespread use. Even an eliminative materialist such as Churchland could not deny that psychotherapy is pragmatic in some clinical situations. So although Churchland (1995, 183) doubted that it is possible to "fix a genuinely broken brain just by talking to it," he wisely wished to avoid imposing on clinical psychiatry a "wholesale replacement of talk therapies with chemical, surgical, and genetic therapies." While Churchland has elaborated philosophical arguments in support of eliminative materialism since the early 1980s, by the mid-1990s (in his book *The Engine of Reason, The Seat of the Soul*) he came to acknowledge the viability of a pragmatically oriented, patient-centered synthesis of clinical neuroscience, psychology, and psychotherapy. This subtle but notable shift in his thinking about the mind/body relation is a testimony to the power of pragmatic reasoning: if unifying scientific theories like eliminative materialism do not serve the practical needs of real people in the real world, then the integrity of those theories is suspect and they will need to be revised accordingly. If clinical psychiatrists—who grapple with the mind/body problem in every interaction with patients—cannot make use of eliminative materialism in clinical practice, then the theory cannot be meaningfully adopted in this practical discipline. And the tenets of philosophical pragmatism would suggest that that consideration must call into serious question the validity and feasibility of eliminative materialism in general.

Despite the impracticality of eliminative materialism, psychiatrists and philosophers of mind ought to remain engaged in scientific reasoning and careful investigation of the role of neuroscience in assessing the effects of psychosocial treatments. Just as renouncing scientific reductionism in psychiatry does not necessarily imply a fall into eclecticism or postmodernism, avoiding eliminative materialism in the philosophy of mind does not necessarily imply a retreat into mysterianism. The pragmatic method can help to rescue both philosophy and psychiatry from extreme and potentially harmful maneuvers. Philosophers and psychiatrists can remain engaged with scientific theory, but avoid the overblown faith in science that is touted by consilience theory or eliminative materialism. Because it is focused on the practical needs of individuals, pragmatism cannot go on faith: it must stay grounded in the scientific evidence and the unique needs of individuals in their everyday lives. Although neuroscience is incomplete, some emerging theories point toward a plausible, clinically oriented conception of mind and brain that adheres to the principles of dialectical pluralism; Kandel's new intellectual framework for psychiatry is one such theory. Pragmatic philosophers and psychiatrists in the twenty-first century must remain open to the development of such scientific theories that usefully address the mind/body problem, even as they recognize the awesome nature of the task and the fact that a science of people is, and will always remain, a multifaceted and open-ended science.

5

Sigmund Freud: Scientist and Pragmatist

Contemporary thinkers like Wilson and Churchland call our attention to shifts from humanistic to scientific explanations in the modern world and to the possibility of further unification of knowledge on the foundation of basic science. A historical perspective on the aspirations of scientists to shift explanations of human behavior from the humanistic to the scientific provides a cautionary tale for our own times. Sigmund Freud's thinking on mind/body issues throughout the early and middle stages of his career is interesting today because it calls attention to the conceivability (and pragmatic necessity) of explanatory shifts in precisely the opposite direction, that is, from the scientific to the humanistic. Freud began his career as a laboratory neuroscientist and yet, for a variety of reasons, later moved in the direction of clinical psychology and psychoanalysis. Tracing some of the twists and turns in Freud's intellectual development on mind/body issues can teach us important lessons regarding the pragmatic nature of psychological explanations and therapies—and shed light on the complicated dialectical relation between neuroscience and psychology—in our own times.

It is worthwhile to study Freud, if only because he too grappled with a vexing science/humanism divide in his career and thought pragmatically about how to overcome it. Although parts of his theory are appropriately in question nowadays, many of his basic psychodynamic principles remain indispensable in the current practice of psychiatry. One can reasonably question the plausibility of many of Freud's most controversial concepts—such as "penis envy" in young girls and "castration anxiety" in young boys—but any serious consideration of clinical psychiatry today cannot overlook the central importance of his ideas and his

reasons for developing the notion of an unconscious mind. Freud introduced and advocated the notion that the human mind is constantly in
conflict with itself and that the individual ego must negotiate the
demands of biological drives such as sexuality and aggression (the id),
the constraints of the moral conscience (the superego), and limitations
imposed by reality. He believed that we structure our experiences and
actions around fears, wishes, and other intrapsychic forces that are
largely outside conscious awareness. When they pursue treatment, people deliver their deepest fears and core emotional conflicts into the psychotherapy setting, where by the process of "transference" they reenact
troubling patterns of relating to important people in their lives—and
over time hopefully rework those patterns in the psychotherapeutic
process. Complex meanings, hidden motives, intrapsychic conflicts,
interpersonal distortions—all part and parcel of human experience and
behavior, and all aspects of the Freudian unconscious—remain some of
the bread and butter issues addressed by psychotherapy today.

The justification for retaining these core Freudian ideas lies not only
in their clinical expediency, but in empirical science as well. Experimental work has suggested that the concept of the unconscious is an important basis for modern cognitive neuroscience. Complicated brain
processes that occur outside awareness are the sine qua non for all conscious thoughts and human activities. In support of this claim,
Westen (2002) offered two cases in point: the "procedural memory" that
allows musicians to play their instruments faster than they can consciously read sheet music, or that allows psychotherapists to respond
empathically to a patient before having developed a consciously articulated formulation of the patient's issues and treatment needs. In such
cases, complex thoughts and emotions are processed quickly and effectively in the absence of concurrent awareness (any awareness of what
happened comes retrospectively, if at all). The existence of unconscious
thoughts and emotional processes has been demonstrated in scores of
research studies reviewed by Westen (1998). For example, in a study of
people with prosopagnosia (a brain disorder that robs the affected person of the capacity to distinguish faces consciously), the investigators
presented pictures of familiar and unfamiliar faces to the subjects while
measuring physiological responses that reflect emotional arousal.

Despite their inability consciously to discriminate the faces they knew from the ones they did not, the subjects had distinct physiological reactions to the two different types of faces, suggesting they could tell the faces apart on an unconscious, emotional level.

The early Freud would have been very interested in attempts by Westen and other cognitive scientists to trace the neuroscientific basis of complex human behavior. In fact, in the early stages of his career, Freud was so engrossed in his work as a neuroscientist that he shared with contemporary eliminative materialists a basic belief that psychological concepts should not figure in rigorous scientific explanations of behavior. Insofar as he hoped to exclude psychological concepts from his methodological armamentarium, Freud in the early stages of his career could be considered a "proto-eliminative materialist." But even though the early Freud can justifiably be described in this way, and despite his early training as a laboratory scientist (and later as a clinical neurologist), he eventually recognized a variety of practical problems with his early position and went on to become the most influential advocate of psychological explanations and treatments in modern history. What considerations underlay Freud's transformation from working as a laboratory scientist (who, like most scientists of his day, denied the existence of unconscious mental life) to becoming a psychoanalyst who believed unconscious mental processes shape human experience and who appreciated the fundamentally dialectical relation of neuroscience and psychology? The pragmatics of clinical explanation and treatment are essential to answering this question.

From the outset of his career, Freud, like some contemporary philosophers and clinical psychiatrists, was an ontological materialist with little tolerance for philosophical symptoms that postulated a transcendent God or a mysterious and disembodied realm of mental life. He came of age at a time when technological advances were increasingly construed as evidence that it would one day become possible to understand the natural world in the terms provided by the physical sciences alone. In keeping with the spirit of the times, Freud assumed a scientific orientation to the world from early in his life (Gay 1988). Throughout his career, he regarded religious doctrines as "illusions and insusceptible of proof" (1927, 31) and rejected explanations of natural events and human actions that appealed to a divine will or immaterial soul. Echoing his demand for a materialistic approach to explaining human behavior, he declared late in his career a basic philosophical view that he consistently had espoused from early on : "Psychoanalysis is a part of science and can adhere to the scientific *Weltanschauung*" (1933, 181).

Several factors motivated the young Freud to cultivate a materialistic worldview. Viennese medicine at the time he enrolled in medical school was dominated by the mechanistic theories of the movement founded by the scientist Hermann Helmholtz in the 1840s. Along with scientists Emil Du Bois–Reymond, Carl Ludwig, and Ernst Brücke, Helmholtz believed that the modern scientist needed to restrict his attention to objectively observable natural phenomena and attempt to formulate rigorous laws that coordinated, explained, and predicted physical events. Like the eliminative materialists today, these members of the "Berlin school" thought all natural phenomena and human behaviors had to be explained in strict accordance with the methods and concepts of the physical sciences. In the paper "Freud's Earliest Theories and the School of Helmholtz," Siegfried Bernfield (1944, 348) traced this history and quoted Du Bois-Reymond, who had made this point unmistakably clear as early as 1842: "No other forces than the common physical chemical ones are active within the organism. In those cases which cannot at the time be explained by these forces one has either to find the specific way or form of their action by means of the physical mathematical model, or to assume new forces equal in dignity to the chemical physical forces inherent in matter, reducible to the force of attraction and repulsion."

It was inevitable that Freud, by enrolling as a medical student in Vienna in the early 1870s, would come under the spell of this scientific tradition. The nature of his early laboratory research reveals the strong hold that Helmholtz's approach had on him. In 1876 Freud did research on the anatomy and physiology of the reproductive organs of male eels and later that year began a 6-year stint as a researcher in Vienna's Institute of Physiology under the supervision of his mentor Brücke. Freud undertook experimental work on the histology of the spinal cord of a primitive fish and conducted microscopic studies of nerve cells of live crayfish. During his years at the Institute of Physiology, he developed a staining method for the microscopic study of nerve tissue and published descriptions of the technique in Viennese medical journals and the British journal *Brain* (1884). After earning a medical degree in 1881, Freud worked at Vienna's Institute of Cerebral Anatomy and authored scientific papers that described the cellular composition of the brain's medulla oblongata. In 1884 he performed a groundbreaking experimental study on the physiological effects of cocaine and in the 1890s published important monographs and textbook chapters on childhood cerebral palsy.

Freud's understanding of the nature of the human mind at this time was guided by the theories of his academic mentors. Not surprisingly, the scientists who trained him regarded mental events as "epiphenomenal" on brain events—that is, brain events caused mental events but mental events caused nothing at all. Their belief was grounded in a profound concern that traditional psychology, with its attention focused on subjective mental experience and imprecise ideas like free will, threatened to undermine the emerging notion of science as empirical study of the mechanical functioning of the natural world. According to this conception, rigorous scientists were in the business of explaining and predicting causally determined events in the natural world, not speculating on the nature of mental processes that were outside the "causal fray." Historian of science Lorraine Daston (1982, 95) noted that there was a pervasive belief among nineteenth-century European scientists that all human behavior needed to be "subordinated to the hegemony of causal—and therefore by implication physiological—explanations." Given that Freud and his mentors considered mental events epiphenomenal and thus excluded psychological concepts from scientific explanations, they can be understood as forerunners of Churchland, or as "proto-eliminative materialists."

Nineteenth-century scientists who worked in the Helmholtzian tradition came to embrace a theory of the mind/body relationship that is best described as "psychophysical parallelism." The proponents of this theory held that any given mental event is necessarily correlated with a describable neurological event, but that the causal arrow pointed only from the physical event to the mental event. They believed, in other words, that the mental depended on and ran in parallel to the neurological, but that it could not interfere causally in the autonomous chain of physical events occurring in the brain. Freud's commitment to keeping neurophysiological and psychological methodologies distinct was consistent with the nature of his early neuroscientific research and its minimization of mental phenomena. By excluding indeterminate psychological concepts like volition from his conceptual vocabulary, Freud could concentrate on investigating and describing neurological processes (whether in eels, crayfish, or human beings) and on demonstrating how these processes obeyed uninterrupted causal laws. His separation of psychological and neurological forms of explanation guaranteed that he could pursue worthwhile scientific research without having to worry that unobservable psychological events might interfere with the causal mechanisms he was trying to elucidate. Thus, in the early stages of his career, Freud held that neurophysiology and psychology represented two distinct explanatory domains running in parallel to one another. Echoing the psychophysical parallelism of the neurologist John Hughlings Jackson (one of Freud's contemporaries), Freud wrote in his monograph *On Aphasia* (1891, 55) that the mental is "a process parallel to the physiological, a 'dependent concomitant.'"

But Freud's mechanistic Helmholtzian background, and his dismissive attitude toward all things mental, had not prepared him adequately for the very practical tasks he began to confront as a physician in the mid-1880s. Viennese medicine at that time, which was steeped in the tradition of Helmholtz, was inept at dealing with clinical presentations that defied neurological laws. Although Freud had become proficient in his ability to localize central nervous system lesions by taking a detailed clinical history and performing a physical examination, his understanding of illnesses that violated well-defined neuroanatomical patterns was rudimentary. He acknowledged that in this stage of his career he was ignorant of the roles played by psychological factors in physical illnesses and that on one especially embarrassing occasion, while he was lecturing to a large medical audience, he misdiagnosed the chronic headaches of a neurotic patient as meningitis. His fellow Viennese physicians, of course, were no more adept than he when explaining and managing such confusing cases. Freud would later write (1925, 12) that his utter disregard in the early 1880s for the psychological dimensions of some clinical disorders was perhaps excusable only because it had "happened at a time when greater authorities than myself in Vienna were in the habit of diagnosing neurasthenia as cerebral tumour."

By the mid-1880s, Freud was seeing more and more of these perplexing cases in his clinical practice. In 1886, for example, he published a report on a hysterical male patient who suffered from left-sided numbness and had several other physical complaints that did not cohere with any identifiable neurological disorder. Freud, unfortunately, was restricted to offering a mere description of the patient's various signs and symptoms, most of which he could not square with any known neurophysiological laws. He certainly had the intuitive sense in this case that psychological factors were relevant to the clinical formulation, because he did describe the patient's bitter financial dispute with his brother that immediately preceded the onset of the symptoms. He further mentioned that during a 2-hour episode that was characterized by "the most violent spasms," the patient kept making reference to that horrific argument with his brother. But without a cogent and pluralistic theory of the mind with which to work, Freud was still in a position to offer a mere clinical description of the patient's physical signs and symptoms, not a convincing account of the multiple factors that caused them.

This case and others like it convinced him that some clinical disorders did not lend themselves to strict neurological explanation. By the late 1880s, Freud had begun to doubt the possibility of excluding psychological concepts from all of his clinical explanations. "There are a large number of patients," Freud (1905b, 284–285) wrote in his paper "Psychical (or Mental) Treatment," "in whom no visible or observable signs of a pathological process can be discovered either during their life or after their death, in spite of all the advances in the methods of investigation made by scientific medicine." His theories no longer cohered with the idea of treating the mind as a mere epiphenomenon of the brain, though it was not until years later in his 1915 paper "The Unconscious" that he explicitly commented on "the insoluble difficulties of psycho-physical parallelism" (p. 168).

Helmholtzian medicine's strict separation of neurology and psychology was clearly hindering progress in the clinical domain. Exhibiting his growing pragmatic sensibility, Freud expressed frustration with the failure of Viennese medicine to account for the confusing clinical pictures seen in illnesses like hysteria and neurasthenia when he reflected in 1887 on "how little the so-called clinical education acquired in our hospitals suffices for the needs of practical physicians" (p. 35). He now became increasingly focused on his inability to understand and treat clinical disorders that seemed to violate the neurological principles he had mastered as a medical student, researcher, and practicing physician in Vienna. Although he would still be referring to the mind as a "dependent concomitant" of the brain as late as 1891, by the mid-1880s Freud already had developed grave worries that the exclusion of psychological concepts from clinical explanations was untenable in many situations. He began to distance himself from his Helmholtzian mentors by writing the following in "Psychical (or Mental) Treatment": "The relationship between the body and the mind is a reciprocal one; but in earlier times the other side of this relation, the effect of the mind upon the body, found little favor in the eyes of physicians. They seemed to be afraid of granting mental life any independence, for fear of that implying an abandonment of the scientific ground on which they stood" (p. 284).

In the first three sections of his landmark 1893 paper contrasting organic and hysterical motor paralyses, Freud limited himself to arguing that hysterical paralyses failed to cohere with any recognizable neuroanatomical patterns. These sections were most likely written in 1888, when Freud was a young clinician who was in the process of realizing that the mechanistic neurology he had been taught in medical school was riddled with explanatory gaps and was failing him when he applied it in the clinic. The fourth and final section of the paper, however, was probably added in 1893 (the publication date for the entire paper), when Freud was already developing a genuinely psychological theory of hysteria. The striking difference between the first three and the fourth sections of the paper prompted James Strachey (1893, 158), the principal editor of Freud's *Standard Edition* in English, to write that this paper constituted "the watershed between Freud's neurological and psychological writings." In the final section, which he added in 1893, Freud wrote that hysterical paralysis could be explained by "an alteration of the *conception*, the *idea*" of the paralyzed region of the body; for pragmatic reasons, he requested "permission to move on to psychological ground—which can scarcely be avoided in dealing with hysteria" (p. 170). Freud now began to argue for the indispensable role of psychology in dealing with clinical challenges presented by hysterical patients: "The signs of their illness originate from nothing other than *a change in the action of their minds upon their bodies* and the immediate cause of their disorders is to be looked for in their minds" (p. 286). Psychophysical parallelism, which held that mental events were causally ineffectual and merely epiphenomenal on brain events, was now rejected because of its pragmatic failure in the clinic.

The pragmatic failures of neuroscience had already been apparent some years earlier to Freud's mentor and colleague Josef Breuer. In late 1880, a 21-year-old Viennese woman named Bertha Pappenheim, now better known by her pseudonym Anna O, had presented to Breuer's medical office complaining of a constellation of physical symptoms that seemed to defy all known patterns of neurological illness. Anna O had initially fallen ill in April of that year during a stressful period when she was nursing her sick father, who had a pulmonary disease that later killed him after a painful and protracted course of illness. Anna O's symptoms included severe cough, double vision, hearing problems, paralysis of her right arm and leg, sensory deficits, lapses of consciousness, and visual hallucinations. Her syndrome was also remarkable for an atypical disturbance of language. When overcome by troubling emotions, for example, she lost her ability to speak or comprehend German (her native tongue) even though she retained her capacity to converse in English. When feeling carefree, on the other hand, she sometimes spoke in French and Italian, and could not remember the times when she was able to speak German and English. During a particularly bizarre episode, Breuer observed that Anna O could somehow read a French text aloud in English but not in French.

There were numerous confusing dimensions to Anna O's presentation. For instance, it openly defied late-nineteenth-century theories of how human language functioning could be altered by disease processes affecting the brain. In keeping with the mainstream neurology of the time, Breuer and Freud thought and worked in accordance with Ribot's law, which stated that pathological changes in the brain of a multilingual individual would only compromise the native language after they had affected the more recently acquired languages (Miller 1991). As

Freud would remark in *On Aphasia* in 1891, "It never happens that an organic lesion causes an impairment affecting the mother tongue and not a later acquired language" (p. 60). Nineteenth-century neurologists believed there could be no exceptions to this elegant "rule of primacy." But Anna O's perplexing language disturbance violated Ribot's law of brain functioning insofar as it was characterized by the cyclical loss and reacquisition of each of the several languages that she spoke.

The disturbing absence of any clear-cut neurological explanation of Anna O's syndrome suggested to Breuer that he had to find an alternative explanation for this bewildering clinical presentation. He concluded that he could only get a grasp on what was happening to her if he entered the domain of psychological explanation. Breuer had learned that he could help Anna O eliminate each of her symptoms in turn by having her talk about them and attempt to recall all of the circumstances that surrounded their initial onset. This cathartic talking process—which Anna O and Breuer called "chimney sweeping"—constituted the first use of Breuer's famous "talking cure." Breuer hypothesized that Anna O's language problems and host of other symptoms were not associated with focal brain lesions but had been caused by psychological traumas, especially those she suffered while caring for her father and witnessing his untimely death. Because Anna O had not been able to articulate her powerful feelings about these traumatic experiences in plain and direct language, they came to be expressed by way of symbolically meaningful physical symptoms and disturbances of her language functioning.

Freud's work would build on the preliminary ideas about psychological causation of symptoms that Breuer began to develop in his treatment of Anna O. Freud recognized in the 1890s that there was a set of patients who suffered from some form of neurological disease (either in the past or in the present) but who at the same time acted in ways that warranted psychological explanations. Despite the fact that their cognition and behavior seemed to be constrained or determined by somatic pathology, it appeared unavoidable to attribute to them a high degree of agency and an ability to adapt their somatic symptoms to serve a variety of psychosocial ends. Some hysterical patients, Freud postulated, were predisposed to developing hysteria because certain parts of their bodies had once been affected by an identifiable physical disease. In 1894, Freud advanced the hypothesis that many such vulnerable individuals possessed a "capacity for conversion," which he described as "a psychophysical aptitude for transposing large sums of excitation into the somatic innervation" (p. 50). He developed the concept of "somatic compliance" in the 1890s to capture his observation that some such people adapt their physical complaints to serve psychological purposes. But he did not formally bestow the name "somatic compliance" on this phenomenon until a decade later, when he wrote (1905a) that susceptible parts of the body often may have psychodynamic meanings "soldered" to them. His theory still has currency: the contemporary theorist Graham Macdonald (1995, 400) argued that "symptoms which are beyond the control of agents—involuntary twitches or tics, say—become neurotic symptoms if used by the agent to express feelings or desire."

Freud brought his theory of somatic compliance into the clinical realm in his treatment of Fräulein Elisabeth von R. (1893–1895), a 24-year-old Viennese woman who for more than 2 years had suffered with crippling leg pains and debilitating fatigue on walking and standing. Her pain was centered mainly in her anterior right thigh with radiation to other areas of her lower extremities, and the skin and muscles of both her lower extremities were hypersensitive to pressure and pinprick. In accordance with the theory of somatic compliance, Freud deemed Elisabeth's legs to be particularly vulnerable because they previously had been affected by rheumatism. "It was probable," Freud wrote, "that an organic change in the muscles was present and that the neurosis attached itself to this and made it seem of exaggerated importance" (p. 138). By probing the content of Elisabeth's feelings and thoughts, Freud discovered a wealth of intriguing clinical material that would help him formulate an integrated psychological and neurological explanation of her illness. He would appeal to both the organic process affecting her lower extremities and to her use of the associated symptoms in psychologically motivated and meaningful ways.

Freud thought Elisabeth's rheumatism predisposed her lower extremities to becoming the focal point of a hysterical disorder, but he also thought that the pains and fatigue she experienced when standing and walking were symbolically meaningful since they served as somatic manifestations of her distressing feelings of helplessness, frustration, and shame, which were brought on by traumatic experiences she had suffered in the past. Freud explained that the initial onset of Elisabeth's hysterical leg weakness could be traced to an experience that was marked by a wrenching conflict between her familial responsibility and her erotic desires. For weeks she had been playing the role of sick-nurse to her ill father, but one night decided to leave him unattended to accompany a boyfriend to a party. Returning home after an evening replete with erotic feelings, she was horrified to learn that her father's condition had badly deteriorated—and she resolved never to go out with her boyfriend again. In so doing, Freud wrote, Elisabeth had repressed her amorous feelings and thoughts from consciousness and had directed the powerful affects associated with them into her legs, which were vulnerable to the development of hysterical symptoms because of the past rheumatic disease.

But it was not only the physical disease affecting Elisabeth's leg muscles that could help to explain why her symptoms had manifested themselves in that particular anatomical distribution. Her symptoms, Freud also hypothesized, were centered in her anterior right thigh because it was in this very area that her sick father used to place his legs every morning while Elisabeth changed his bandages. Freud referred to this part of her body, now invested with symbolic meaning that was related to the emotional trauma of sick-nursing, as an "artificial hysterogenic zone." Freud believed that her leg pains, like the hysterical symptoms he observed in so many of his patients, served a wide variety of ends and contained so many meanings that he referred to them as psychologically "overdetermined." He noted that Elisabeth's leg pains upon standing also revealed her deep unhappiness about "standing alone" in the world, in painful contrast to her happily married sister. The leg pains also symbolized Elisabeth's helpless sense that she could not "take a single step forward" toward the restoration of her previous happiness or that of her family. Effective treatment of a patient like Elisabeth, Freud discovered, would require more than just attending to her rheumatism. It would also involve helping her understand, articulate, and work through the overwhelming emotions that were underlying (and being expressed through) her physical symptoms.

Freud dealt with other clinical cases in the early- and mid-1890s that presented practical challenges akin to Elisabeth's leg pains, including the facial pains (neuralgia) of his patient Frau Cäcilie M (1893). Cäcilie, according to Freud's report, had suffered on and off since childhood from a neuralgia of two branches of her trigeminal nerve, which innervates the face. Because the cause of the neuralgia was thought by medical consultants to be gout, she frequently received the standard treatment of "the electric brush, alkaline water, and purges" (p. 176). She had received radical dental surgery years earlier when it was suspected that the source of her recurrent trigeminal neuralgia resided in the roots of her teeth. Freud's theory of somatic compliance, of course, suggested that in adulthood her face would be susceptible to developing hysterical symptoms. Hysterical facial pains, Freud pointed out, first became apparent during an episode when her husband made a remark that she interpreted as a mortal insult. She said that her husband's comment had felt like "a slap in the face," leading Freud (1893, 179) to hypothesize that by symbolization she had adapted her facial pain to serve a psychological purpose. "A whole set of physical sensations which would ordinarily be regarded as organically determined," Freud (1893, 180) wrote, "were in her case of psychical origin or at least possessed a psychical meaning." As a pragmatist, Freud realized that any effective treatment of the facial neuralgia would have to go beyond the standard treatment regimen for gout and be directed at the psychological and interpersonal uses that she made of her facial pain.

Freud's appreciation of the importance of psychological explanations was not ivory-tower theorizing about the mind and its pathologies. Freud, instead, was a pragmatic thinker who, from the mid-1880s onward, was continuously engaged in clinical work with patients like Elisabeth, who had come to him for the relief of symptoms that were extremely real and painful to them. He needed a theory that was clinically informed and could be applied to help patients who were suffering. By fits and starts, Freud came to think that his psychoanalytic techniques could be implemented in such a way as to help certain patients live a happier and more autonomous existence. In several papers on psychoanalytic technique, published between 1911 and 1915, Freud focused his attention on providing other clinicians with practical advice on how to conduct a psychotherapy or psychoanalysis that was in the best interest of the patient. But it was several years earlier that Freud first had realized that psychoanalytic explanations of some patients' illnesses could lead to effective therapies unavailable to physicians practicing in strict accordance with the precepts of nineteenth-century Helmholtzian medicine.

There is little dispute that many of the therapies Freud recommended to patients in the early part of his career—such as hypnosis and hydrotherapy—were in most cases ineffective. Likewise, the standard medical treatments of diseases such as Cäcilie's gout—which included "the electric brush, alkaline water, and purges"—were largely unsuccessful. Recognizing this fact, Freud remarked in his paper on psychoanalytic technique titled "Observations on Transference-Love" (1915a) that "to believe that the psychoneuroses are to be conquered by operating with harmless little remedies is grossly to underestimate those disorders both as to their origins and their practical importance" (p. 171). During the 1880s, Freud and Breuer became keenly aware of the need for therapeutic approaches that might succeed where Helmholtzian medicine failed. It was this very awareness that motivated Breuer in 1880 to undertake a "talking cure" of Anna O's hysteria. Despite his statements to the contrary, Breuer failed in his attempt to effect a lasting cure for Anna O. But by the early years of the twentieth century, Freud's psychoanalytic technique had matured to a degree that he could now reflect on Breuer's earlier blunders and suggest how future clinicians might avoid the practical pitfalls that his clinical mentor had encountered years before in that particularly challenging case.

In "Observations on Transference-Love," Freud suggested that the core problem that plagued Anna O's course of treatment was Breuer's failure to understand that she had fallen in love with him and had developed a fantasy of giving birth to his baby. Freud believed that this astonishing development had been a clear example of "transference," a process by which a patient experiences and acts toward the psychoanalyst as though the latter were a representation of a person (or persons) who had played a critical role in the early development of the former. Anna O's falling in love with Breuer, in particular, could be understood as a transference of powerful feelings of affection for her father onto Breuer, who came to serve as a vehicle through which she could "act out" her intense (and primarily unconscious) feelings. Freud warned clinicians that a patient's falling in love with the analyst is usually a result of transference and not of any virtues the analyst may possess. Breuer, unfortunately, was clearly unable to grasp the significance of Anna O's transference-love during the time he worked with her between 1880 and 1882. In his "On the History of the Psychoanalytic Movement" (1914a), Freud criticized Breuer for regarding her hysterical pregnancy as merely an "untoward event" and for terminating her psychotherapy abruptly in the context of an intensification of her transference-love. The absence of a working concept of unconscious fantasy and motivation had led to an undesirable practical outcome in Anna O's case.

While he described techniques the analyst could use to handle pathological transferences and to avoid clinical disasters such as the termination of treatment (as finally occurred in the case of Anna O), Freud also believed that under most circumstances the transference could be incorporated as a useful dimension of the treatment process. In his essay on technique titled "Remembering, Repeating, and Working-Through" (1914b), Freud noted that a patient can derive therapeutic benefit by grappling with the transference in the context of a good psychoanalytic therapy. By allowing the patient to effect a transference of thoughts and feelings stemming from past events and relationships onto the clinician, and encouraging the patient to reflect on the nature and dynamics of that transference, the clinician could help the patient attain a greater degree of insight into past life events and present-day motivations, thereby helping him or her gain greater freedom and mastery with respect to overwhelming feelings, thoughts, and behaviors. The "transference-neurosis" created in psychoanalysis, in other words, was similar to the real-life neurosis the patient experienced but, as Freud pointed out, it was also "accessible to our intervention"—which is to say it could be worked through and transformed. The activity of working through transference became the cornerstone of Freud's mature psychoanalytic technique and it remains so in many versions of contemporary psychodynamic psychotherapy. As he wrote in "Observations on Transference-Love," the psychotherapy setting can serve as a "playground" where the patient can explore ways to overcome troubling and compulsive patterns. Working through the transference became an important psychoanalytic technique not for theoretical reasons, but because it worked in a pragmatic sense.

Having learned that some illnesses were best treated by working through the transference-neurosis, Freud (1915a, 171) wrote that some patients require a "psychoanalysis which is not afraid to handle the most dangerous mental impulses and to obtain mastery over them for the benefit of the patient."

Freud's maturing psychoanalytic technique can be seen at work in his treatment of the obsessional neurosis of his 29-year-old patient known as the Ratman (1909) because of his troubling obsession that his father and a "lady friend" were victims of a cruel torture whereby rats bored into their anuses. The Ratman's irrational thoughts and behaviors, Freud suggested, were the result of primitive unconscious fantasies that reflected his unarticulated feelings of love and hatred for significant people in his life. In a telling incident Freud reported, the Ratman removed a stone from the road over which his lady friend's carriage was about to pass—an act by which he expressed affection and concern for her. By replacing the stone in the middle of the road a few moments later, however, he revealed his hostile and resentful feelings toward his lady friend, who was unable to bear children and whom the Ratman therefore regarded as an undesirable spouse. As he repeatedly and compulsively removed and replaced the stone in her path, the Ratman did not yet understand that he was acting out an unconscious fantasy of derision and rage toward someone for whom he also harbored loving, tender feelings. Lacking insight into the malicious nature of his replacing the stone in the middle of the road, the Ratman told Freud that he had done this simply because he realized how absurd it had been to have removed the stone in the first place. This rationalization suggested to Freud that the Ratman lacked the capacity to tolerate ambivalent feelings or to articulate simultaneous feelings of love and hatred for one and the same person.

During his time in psychoanalysis, the Ratman gradually became more and more aware of the repressed hatred he had for his father and his lady friend—as well as for Freud, on whom he now acted out his deep-seated conflict between love and hate "along the painful road of transference." In the course of treatment, the Ratman's transference was increasingly characterized by aggressive impulses toward Freud and, in response to these impulses, self-reproaches for his ostensibly senseless feelings. At one critical juncture, he roamed Freud's consulting room describing his fantasies and then cowered before Freud as though Freud were about to give him a beating. He rationalized his behavior by saying that he could not report such distressing thoughts and fantasies while reclining comfortably on a couch. But this rationalization was unconvincing even to himself, and he soon found "a more cogent explanation" of his odd behavior: he was afraid that Freud would punish him for committing sexual indiscretions. Although the Ratman did not consciously believe that Freud was his real father about to beat him for these misdeeds, he seemed to elaborate this fantasy because his mind was structured to perceive male authority figures as the sources of sexual prohibition—akin to a prohibition against masturbation his father had lain on him in early childhood. The transference fantasy of Freud-as-father is intelligible when it is understood that, in the words of Freud (1909, 200), "The conflict at the root of his illness was in essentials a struggle between the persisting influence of his father's wishes and his own amatory predilections."

The Ratman's treatment with Freud afforded him an opportunity for the kind of self-examination that would empower him to acquire greater mastery of the unconscious conflicts that were dominating his life and compromising his intimate relationships. He came to recognize that his seemingly unintelligible actions resulted in part from his fantasies of people placing barriers to his erotic fulfillment, and from his own valiant but misdirected attempts to overcome these barriers. As the Ratman came to realize that his love and hatred for his father structured all of his later relationships and impelled him to irrational and self-destructive actions, he acquired a growing capacity to judge each relationship on its own terms. At first, the Ratman was only able to act out his primitive and aggressive feelings toward his father, but the exploration of his transference of hateful feelings for his father onto Freud provided him with the opportunity to begin to transform these overwhelming unconscious fantasies into manageable thoughts, judgments, and actions. Freud (1909, 228) came to realize that favorable practical outcomes for certain neurotic patients like the Ratman depended on a treatment that "traces their unconscious thoughts and translates them into conscious ones."

By recognizing the utility of psychological explanations to guide certain treatments such as that of the Ratman, Freud made possible the wide range of psychotherapies used effectively today. These therapies include the psychodynamic and psychoanalytic approaches that grew directly out of Freud's clinical work. But they also include the cognitive-behavioral therapies (CBT) that are rooted in the idea that self-critical thinking (and other pathological forms of thinking) can cause mental disorders, and that these disorders are best treated in a psychotherapy process that challenges and restructures that pattern of thinking. At the same time, Freud always remained modest about the power of his technique to help patients make thoroughgoing changes and, in keeping with his pragmatic sensibility, he recognized the provisional nature of all psychological achievements that may occur in psychotherapy. In a late paper titled "Analysis Terminable and Interminable," Freud (1937, 248) wrote that psychoanalysis can be understood as one of the "'impossible' professions in which one can be sure beforehand of achieving unsatisfying results." So how does one know when a patient's psychoanalysis is complete and can be terminated? The answer to that question, Freud believed, could not be determined on theoretical grounds because it was a purely "practical matter":

It is not easy to foresee a natural end, even if one avoids any exaggerated expectations and sets the analysis no excessive tasks. Our aim will not be to rub off every peculiarity of human character for the sake of a schematic "normality," nor yet to demand that the person who has been "thoroughly analysed" shall feel no passions and develop no internal conflicts. The business of the analysis is to secure the best possible psychological conditions for the functions of the ego; with that it has discharged its task (p. 250).

Freud's pragmatism manifested itself in his deep concern for favorable practical outcomes for patients and in his provisional sensibility about clinical formulations and treatments. This pragmatic sensibility remains relevant to contemporary psychotherapy and psychoanalysis, in which there has been a growing movement toward giving greater priority to clinical outcomes than to rigid adherence to theory and technique. In the article "The Tendency to Neglect Therapeutic Aims in Psychoanalysis," psychoanalyst Michael Bader (1994) critiqued the field's long-standing tendency to value strictly defined goals and techniques of the psychoanalytic process (such as psychological interpretations aimed at fostering insight and self-awareness) above the patients' own wishes and desires to feel better rather than understand themselves in depth. Achievement of greater self-understanding certainly can help some individuals feel better in the course of psychotherapy or psychoanalysis, but the decision to pursue insight-oriented treatment needs to be negotiated between patient and clinician, not imposed by a clinician working with a doctrinaire set of theories and techniques. Most patients consider the pursuit of psychological insight worthwhile only if it leads them to feel and function better in their everyday lives. As a clinical enterprise, psychoanalysis must aim to have a practical impact rather than to define and strictly adhere to an inflexible theory and methodology.

Therefore, psychotherapists and psychoanalysts constantly face the challenge of having to work pragmatically in the dialectical space between adherence to strict theory and technique and application of their own creativity, personal styles, and capacities to connect empathically with their individual patients. Freud's interests in the practicalities of patient care, development of large-scale theories of human mental life, and description of his psychoanalytic technique required a capacity for multidimensional and dialectical reasoning. More so than ever, the contemporary clinician also must be able to reason and work dialectically and pragmatically. In the article "Dialectical Thinking and Therapeutic Action in the Psychoanalytic Process," psychoanalyst Irwin Hoffman (1994, 200–201) encouraged the clinician to maintain a flexible and provisional stance when negotiating the dialectic of adherence to strict technique and expression of one's own creativity:

The fact that analysts cannot know exactly how they should position themselves with respect to the dialectic of overtly expressive participation and relatively standard, authority-enhancing technique is precisely the wellspring for an overarchingly authentic way of being with the patient, one that is marked by a sense of struggle with uncertainty, by a willingness to "play it both ways," and by an openness to consideration of the unconscious meanings, for the analyst and the patient, of whatever course has been taken.

Finally, Freud's pragmatism also manifested itself in his dialectical pluralism. Even as Freud developed psychoanalysis and advocated for the practicality of psychological explanations, he never abandoned his hopes for refining scientific approaches to understanding the human experience. Instead, he remained open to the possibility that future neuroscientific discoveries would add to our growing knowledge about human psychology and possibly even guide us to reconceptualize our entire structure of beliefs about human behavior. In 1915 he wrote that "our psychical topography has *for the present* nothing to do with anatomy" (1915b, 175)—and yet in 1920 he speculated that any remaining problems in the psychoanalytic understanding of human beings "would probably vanish if we were already in a position to replace the psychological terms by physiological or chemical ones" (p. 60). Until the time he died in 1939, Freud believed that mental life depends on complex brain functioning, that greater understanding of the brain could lead us to rework our understanding of human psychology, and that in the meantime—while the nature of the complex interaction between the physical brain and the meaningful mind remains shrouded in mystery, and psychiatric science remains incomplete—clinicians must use a multitude of explanatory concepts and treatment methodologies to do all they can to help ease their patients' suffering.

Freud's legacy lives on in the twenty-first century, largely because of his pragmatic approach to understanding and treating his patients. His move from neurology to psychology early in his career was driven by practical considerations in the context of the failure of traditional Helmholtzian medical science to guide appropriate treatment of complex patients whose illnesses were shaped by their motivations, emotions, and interpersonal situations. Once he committed himself wholeheartedly to the challenges of human psychology, his theory and technique continued to evolve in the face of practical considerations. His refinements of his clinical technique, and his emphasis on the use of the transference-neurosis to promote desirable clinical changes, suggest that his thinking about the human mind was heavily influenced by an abiding commitment to help people whose minds were tormented by anxiety and other forms of suffering. At the same time, Freud retained a pluralistic and provisional view of the human experience, and a hopeful open-mindedness to the possibility that future scientific advances would tell us something new about ourselves and might even lead us to rethink the very foundations of the human sciences. These values and principles, rooted in the challenges and realities of Freud's clinical encounters decades ago, continue to guide the pragmatic psychiatrist today.

6

Pragmatism in Neurology and Psychiatry

Over the course of his career, Freud moved farther and farther away from laboratory neuroscience and clinical neurology, and immersed himself more and more in the details of clinical psychology. But with the continuous expansion of neuroscience in our own time, clinicians are faced again with concerns about the complicated nature of the relation between neurology and psychiatry. Advances in neuroscience continue to enhance the understanding and treatment of neurological and psychiatric disorders. This fact has prompted some physicians to entertain the possibility that neurology and psychiatry eventually can merge into one discipline that rests on the foundation of clinical neuroscience. Other physicians view the relationship between neurology and psychiatry very differently. Regardless of how far neuroscience may advance in the near or long-term future, they argue, clinical psychiatry ought to remain an autonomous discipline. This debate about defining the appropriate relationship between the two major medical disciplines addressing complex human experience and behavior has important theoretical and practical dimensions.

Clinical pragmatism has something to add to this debate. The foundational science of clinical neurology always has been (and remains) neuroscience, but the same cannot be said of psychiatry, which has numerous foundational sciences—ranging from basic neuroscience to the social sciences and humanities. Because neurology and psychiatry ground themselves in overlapping but distinct concepts that are necessary to provide effective care to a broad spectrum of patients, they should not merge now or at any time in the future. Most neurological disorders are caused by lesions and functional aberrations of the central and peripheral nervous systems, but psychiatric disorders tend to be caused by multiple factors, including neurological, intrapsychic, and interpersonal problems. Moreover, while treatment of neurological disorders is somatic in nature, treatment of psychiatric illness may include somatic modalities (such as psychopharmacology and ECT) but often cannot be limited to such modalities. Psychotherapies and psychosocial approaches are critical aspects of psychiatric treatment and in most cases could not be replaced by purely somatic approaches without seriously compromising the practical benefits of treatment.

Among the primary conceptual and practical distinctions between clinical neurology and clinical psychiatry is their fundamentally different view of the nature of symptoms. Neurologists understand sensory, motor, and behavioral symptoms as the result of lesions in the brain or other components of the human nervous system. The rationale for their approach is clear and sound, whether we are considering disorders of the central or peripheral nervous system. Abnormal electrical discharges in the brain are the clear cause of seizures. Damage to motor neurons in the spinal cord is the undisputed cause of amyotrophic lateral sclerosis (also known as Lou Gehrig's disease), a devastating disorder characterized by progressive muscle atrophy and breathing problems. A well-defined genetic abnormality is the accepted cause of neuropsychiatric impairments in patients with Huntington's disease. The mechanistic notion of cause and effect in neurology is supported by empirical evidence, such as that provided by genetic tests, electroencephalography (EEG), and postmortem study of brain tissue. It is also justified by the success of treatments grounded in this understanding, such as the use of anticonvulsant medications to prevent seizures. The nature of causation in clinical neurology is straightforward and elegant: lesions in the nervous system cause observable clinical syndromes that require somatic therapy. The syndromes are neither adaptive nor meaningful: they just happen to people and they represent undesirable, unfortunate, and sometimes debilitating and life-threatening events for the affected individuals.

Similarly, symptoms in certain psychiatric disorders result primarily from neurological insults, as in cases of major depression associated with Huntington's disease or following a left-sided brain stroke, musical hallucinations associated with a pathological process in the left temporal lobe, personality changes due to temporal lobe epilepsy, and disinhibited behavior resulting from Alzheimer's dementia or an injury to the orbitofrontal region of the brain. The emergence of a robust neuropsychiatry over the last few decades, beginning with the influential work of the behavioral neurologist Norman Geschwind (1975), has increased awareness of the neurological causation of numerous psychiatric disorders. But the causation of other (and perhaps most) mental disorders is murkier and more complex. Some individuals have a genetic predisposition to mood disorders (as evidenced by a strong family history of these illnesses) but actually become depressed only in the context of stressful life events. Some patients communicate disavowed anger or repressed fear of an impending challenge by slipping into a depressed state. Psychiatrist Randolph Nesse (2000, 14) wrote that major depression can serve adaptive purposes, such as "communicating a need for help, signaling yielding in a hierarchy conflict, fostering disengagement from commitments to unreachable goals, and regulating patterns of investment."

Likewise, some individuals with a biological predisposition to mood instability or bipolar disorder may become manic in order to flee an unbearable interpersonal situation, such as a faltering career or a failing marriage. Other individuals with a predisposition to psychotic disorders (such as schizophrenia) may develop delusional ideas that serve to distance them from a painful reality and to enhance their self-esteem and sense of purpose. Psychoanalyst Martin Willick (1993, 1137) pointed out that although schizophrenia clearly is associated with major derangements in brain function, its clinical features derive from complex interactions among "the basic biological abnormalities, the methods used to cope with these abnormalities, the degree of ego integration that preceded the onset of the illness, the particular dynamic conflicts in each patient, and a multitude of stresses in the environmental milieu." As described in chapter 3, Adam's delusion about fulfilling the mission of Billie Holiday appeared to result from his brain dysfunction in combination with his wish to lend meaning to his emotional suffering. Clinical material and published literature discussed later in this chapter also support the idea that psychiatric disorders, unlike neurological disorders, may have multiple causes spanning the biopsychosocial spectrum and be imbued with profound existential and interpersonal meaning.

Proponents of merging neurology and psychiatry argue that both disciplines ought to regard neuroscience as their principal foundation. In a paper titled "Neurology and Psychiatry: Closing the Great Divide," which was the lead article in the journal *Neurology* in January 2000 (Price, Adams, and Coyle 2000, 12), two neurologists and a psychiatrist argued that the "explosion of neuroscientific knowledge has rendered the traditional boundaries between neurology and psychiatry increasingly indistinct." In another paper titled "The Integration of Neurology, Psychiatry, and Neuroscience in the 21st Century," neurologist Joseph Martin (2002, 695) wrote that "the interests of neurology and psychiatry converge within the framework of modern neuroscience." Considering the exciting and compelling neuroscientific research on the brain processes that are correlated with many psychological processes and mental disorders, these claims are not without merit. But clinicians and theorists who favor a full-blown merger of neurology and psychiatry tend either to overlook or undervalue the importance of psychosocial causation of mental disorders and the adaptive, purposive, and meaningful nature of psychiatric symptoms.

The constriction of (or complete disregard for) psychosocial causation, adaptive functioning, and meaning of psychiatric symptoms, however, flies in the face of both empirical research and widely held philosophical assumptions about human behavior. There is empirical evidence not only that stressful life events can contribute to the causation of major depressive episodes (Kendler, Karkowski, and Prescott 1999), but also that delusions may be caused in part by psychological factors (Roberts 1991) and that high levels of expressed emotion in family contexts may exacerbate the symptomatic course of schizophrenia (Leff and Vaughn 1985). There is, moreover, extensive literature on various social factors that can contribute to the causation of mental illnesses (Eisenberg 1995). In addition, research in cognitive neuroscience has suggested that mental states are not merely epiphenomenal on neuronal states but in fact play important causal roles. On this topic, a book by psychologist Derek Bolton and psychiatrist Jonathan Hill (1996) delineated the causal role of mental events in psychiatry and psychology. In one of Bolton's papers (1997, 264), he wrote simply that "explanations in terms of meaning are to be regarded as just as causal, and just as much a part of science, as explanations in terms of physical or chemical lesions." He is joined by numerous philosophers of mind who believe in mental causation (Corbí and Prades 2000; Putnam 1999) and by psychiatrists who argue that the meaningful dimensions of personal experience can determine the nature and course of mental disorder as much as the neuroscientific dimensions can (Gabbard 1992; Frattaroli 2001).

Other philosophers and psychiatrists take this argument a step further by emphasizing the impossibility of conceptualizing neurological causation in the absence of a meaningful human "life world" in which such causation acquires context and relevance. Psychiatrist Michael Schwartz and philosopher Osborne Wiggins (1985, 339) argued that "everyday experience constitutes the fundamental context that bestows meaning even on those activities that go beyond it," such as basic neuroscience. Without a "prescientific" life world to lend it context and meaning, basic neuroscience is just an abstract pursuit that has little practical applicability in clinical settings. Considered in this way, it is debatable whether basic neuroscience could even qualify as the foundational science of clinical neurology, which, as a practical discipline, grounds itself in the ordinary human life world. The case against neuroscience as foundational is even more convincing and robust in psychiatry, where symptoms are understood to have existential meaning and to serve important social ends in the life world. The abstractions of neuroscience cannot encompass the pragmatics of psychiatric explanation and treatment, which must embrace the humanistic notions of psychosocial meaning and adaptation.

The pragmatic point of view is indispensable here. Clinical pragmatism is a central operating principle in psychiatry and ought to be front and center as psychiatrists grapple with both the scientific and humanistic complexities of psychiatric explanation. From the standpoint of the pragmatically oriented clinician, the goal of exploring the question of whether neurology and psychiatry should merge is to fine-tune our diagnostic and therapeutic methodologies for the sake of enhancing patient care. In this debate on how best to define the relations among psychiatry, neurology, and neuroscience, we must ask what is at stake for real-world patients who present to hospitals, clinics, and consulting rooms seeking relief from their suffering. Deliberations about whether the disciplines should merge or remain separate cannot be divorced from considerations of the practical effects of these deliberations on the nature and quality of the clinical care that individuals receive.

Discussion of particular psychiatric syndromes and clinical cases can help to demonstrate the impracticality of regarding neuroscience as the sole foundation of psychiatry. Psychogenic seizures provide a case in point. How are clinicians to explain and treat seizures that occur in the absence of a clear neurological cause? A psychogenic seizure has been defined as "an observable abrupt change in consciousness or behavior that was not due to a known physiologic cause or accompanied by an ictal or postictal alteration in the EEG" (Leis, Ross, and Summers 1992, 95). The standard method that neurologists currently employ to distinguish epileptic and psychogenic seizures is video-EEG testing in specialized hospital centers, in which the patient gets monitored continuously over several hours for evidence of simultaneous epileptic changes observed on EEG and convulsive motor activity recorded on videotape. If the latter occurs in the absence of the former, then the diagnosis of psychogenic seizures is made with a reasonable degree of diagnostic certainty. Although it is employed less routinely, the more sophisticated (though physically invasive) method of implanting electrodes deep inside the relevant parts of the patient's brain allows for more sensitive testing to determine whether the patient is experiencing epileptic seizure activity.

Contemporary neurologists have observed that there are numerous clinical markers that might further help to distinguish epileptic and psychogenic seizures. Some investigators, for example, have reported that blood levels of the hormone prolactin are significantly elevated immediately after the occurrence of epileptic seizures but not after psychogenic seizures. Many neurologists believe that by employing enhanced EEG, neuroimaging, and laboratory techniques that will undoubtedly become available in the years to come, it is conceivable that all forms of seizures—including the ones currently diagnosed as psychogenic—will be understandable in terms of brain disease. It has already been suggested that epileptic seizures that originate in the brain's frontal lobe can cause many of the very same symptoms that are widely believed to be associated with psychogenic seizures, such as pelvic thrusting and side-to-side head movements (Saygi et al. 1992). Here is another example of how somatic symptoms that once appeared to require psychological explanation may yield to strictly neurological explanation. It is conceivable that neurologists in the twenty-first century will learn that the behaviors currently described as psychogenic seizures are actually epileptic seizures that at one time were clinically undetectable. Such a finding would strengthen the argument that neurology and psychiatry can and ought to merge.

But countervailing evidence suggests that some psychogenic seizures cannot be adequately understood or pragmatically treated without introducing a robust notion of unconscious motivation and communication. Psychiatrists have pointed out that psychogenic seizures usually occur in the daytime, in a state of full wakefulness, and in the presence of an audience (Roy 1989). Some clinicians have claimed that patients' vocalizations during psychogenic seizures are often characterized by "an emotional flavor suggestive of crying or feeling pain" (Saygi et al. 1992, 1275). Consistent with Freud's idea that hysterical symptoms violate strict neuroanatomical laws, some clinicians have observed that psychogenic seizures are marked by the "nonphysiologic spread of neurologic signs" (Chabolla et al. 1996, 496). Improvements in diagnostic technologies might allow clinicians to explain these events in terms of associated brain changes, and better psychotropic drugs might help to prevent these events in some patients. Nonetheless, psychogenic seizures may allow patients to express distress and to seek psychological help when they are unable to tolerate painful and overwhelming emotions that they cannot articulate and that may be related to a traumatic event or an interpersonal challenge. Some patients who have histories of well-documented epileptic seizures also go on to have psychogenic seizures that are not associated with clear EEG abnormalities and that appear to convey otherwise unexpressed emotions such as anger, fear, or sexual desire. No advance in scientific neurology would ever allow clinicians to avoid grappling with the intrapsychic and interpersonal dynamics of such patients. And to ensure that such patients receive pluralistic care that dialectically synthesizes neurological, psychological, and interpersonal aspects of the case, psychiatry ought to remain a separate discipline.

Panic disorder is another case in point. Some researchers have argued that the three phases of panic disorder—the acute panic attack, anticipatory anxiety of having another panic attack, and phobic avoidance of situations where the attacks may occur—can be explained on the basis of abnormal neuronal excitation in three interconnected brain regions: the brain stem, limbic system, and prefrontal cortex (Gorman et al. 1989). Support for this claim comes in part from empirical findings that infusions of panic-inducing pharmacological agents (such as sodium lactate and yohimbine) increase firing rates of certain neurons in the brain stem's locus ceruleus, while agents that prevent panic attacks (such as imipramine and clonidine) reduce those firing rates. Others who study panic disorder, however, oppose the idea that it can be accounted for on a purely neuroscientific basis. Cognitive-behavioral theorists, for example, have argued that panic attacks are often caused by a patient's "catastrophic misinterpretation" of somatic sensations like mild chest pain and shortness of breath (Busch et al. 1991). Psychodynamic theorists go on to ask why some individuals misinterpret their bodily sensations in the first place and suggest that such sensations often have unconscious meaning—and that misinterpretations of those sensations can serve useful purposes. Panic attacks may be psychologically motivated responses to unconscious fears of isolation, separation, entrapment, or other threats (Busch et al. 1991). "In some cases anxiety may reflect an apparently random electrochemical burst from the locus ceruleus," wrote psychiatrist Glen Gabbard (1992, 996). "In other cases anxiety may serve as a window on unconscious conflict."

Panic disorder is one of many diagnostic entities in psychiatry for which there is no broadly accepted explanatory model. In the absence of a consensual approach to explaining and treating it, clinicians ought to take an open-minded, provisional, and pragmatically oriented approach. Psychiatrist Barbara Milrod and her colleagues (1996) described a case in which she did just that. The patient, Ms. A, was an educated young woman with a history since the second grade of panic attacks marked by rapid heartbeat and breathing, loss of balance, and a sense of doom. She had had a chaotic childhood in which she felt ignored and abandoned by her father (who had severe bipolar disorder) and suffered separation anxiety vis-à-vis her mother (who had survived

Nazi concentration camps). Milrod and her colleagues explained that Ms. A declined psychotropic medication for her panic disorder, because it evoked unpleasant memories of her father's psychiatric illness and his use of lithium to control it. Ms. A also resisted the suggestion of formal cognitive-behavioral therapy, because she took the suggestion to imply that she was not bright enough to engage in insight-oriented psychotherapy. Milrod flexibly and pragmatically embarked on a course of psychodynamic therapy in which Ms. A's exploration of complex transference issues empowered her to take control of her symptoms by acquiring insight into her anger and profound fear of separation and abandonment. "This enabled her to relinquish her panic attacks," Milrod and her colleagues wrote, "which to her represented a somatic, masochistic communication of her rage and sense of isolation" (p. 700). A clinical neurologist operating only with neuroscience as a foundation would not have had the conceptual or clinical tools to provide Ms. A with such effective treatment. Even if a neuroscientist could identify a plausible biological cause of Ms. A's condition, a pragmatically oriented psychiatrist would still need a psychological approach to provide her with any therapeutic benefit.

Another case that highlights the inadequacy of exclusively neuroscientific reasoning in psychiatry is that of my patient named Cara, who had a long-standing history of catatonic depression and medical problems such as hypothyroidism. Her catatonic episodes (characterized by a severely depressed mood, anorexia, mutism, and muscle rigidity) apparently had a neurological cause given her good response to ECT, thyroid replacement therapy, and psychotropic medications, including antidepressants. However, Cara required more frequent ECT and higher medication doses in the aftermath of a traumatic experience with a social worker who tried to explore some of Cara's painful childhood memories of being beaten by her father. This ill-fated therapy was terminated when it was discovered that Cara's catatonic depression likely had been exacerbated by the social worker's unsolicited attempt to have Cara confront memories and emotions she was unable to tolerate. It was plausible that Cara became more catatonic in order to avoid a painful and overwhelming confrontation with terrifying but repressed memories of child abuse.

While Cara's catatonic depression clearly had neurological under-pinnings, it was helpful to take psychological factors into account in order to explain the timing, severity, meaning, and adaptive nature of her clinical exacerbation—and to make the sound therapeutic decision to discontinue exploratory psychotherapy with the social worker (but to continue more supportive psychotherapy with a different clinician). This case illustrates the role of integrating a pluralistic set of concepts that span the biopsychosocial spectrum in order to ensure pragmati-cally grounded patient care. A merger of neurology and psychiatry on the reductive foundation of neuroscience would not have allowed for this multifaceted and pragmatic explanation and course of action. Although Cara's treatment became predominantly somatic in nature (i.e., ongoing ECT and medication treatment), psychiatric reasoning helped to explain the fluctuations in her clinical state and to consider if and when it might ever be helpful to explore her emotionally charged memories and thoughts from childhood. The pragmatic focus on achieving the best outcome for Cara led to a psychological explanation of her catatonic episode and a predominantly somatic approach to treating it.

Another narrative that reveals the failure of neuroscience to fully ground clinical psychiatry, reported by psychiatrist Edward Hundert (1992), is that of a patient named Tim, a young man with the delusion that he was the reincarnation of Hitler and was placed on Earth to do penance for his crimes against humanity. At age 10 Tim had suffered a severe head injury with loss of consciousness and at age 12 had been diagnosed with multiple sclerosis (MS), a waxing and waning neurolog-ical disorder that causes weakness and sensory deficits. At age 20 he had started to have recurrent episodes of depression, paranoia, social with-drawal, and impulsivity, including several nearly fatal suicide attempts. Following a suicide attempt at age 23, Tim had begun to believe that he had committed a blasphemous act in trying to take his own life. Shortly thereafter, he developed his elaborate delusional scheme, which included the inalterable belief that he had been buried alive in Hitler's grave for 5 years and had then come back to life to suffer for Hitler's crimes. Magnetic resonance imaging (MRI) of Tim's brain at that time revealed numerous lesions in white-matter regions of his brain, though it was unclear whether the lesions were associated primarily with the childhood head injury or with an MS exacerbation.

There is sound neuropsychiatric evidence that MS is highly associated with mood disorders (such as depression and bipolar disorder) and that affective illnesses are generally more severe in patients who have MS than in comparison patients who do not (Lyoo et al. 1996). Such evidence includes the MS patients' lengthier hospital stays, more frequent admissions, and greater requirement for psychiatric medications after discharge. Aware of the correlation between MS and behavioral disorders, Hundert noted that in Tim's case, it would be "tempting to assume that the brain pathology which lights up so clearly on his MRI scan is the direct cause of his fixed belief" (p. 348). However, the content of Tim's delusion—the details about Hitler—cannot be understood in biological terms but can be made intelligible only in terms of Tim's life story. An individual with the same brain lesions from a different culture or period in history probably would have had a delusion as well, but the content of that person's delusion might not have had anything to do with Hitler. Even in this case where brain pathology indicated a likely cause of the delusion, only meaningful psychology could elucidate the delusion's actual content. The idea that psychological explanation can be relevant in a clinical setting in which the importance of brain-based causal explanation is also so undeniable suggests serious problems for strict biological reductionism and the project to merge neurology and psychiatry.

The work of the early- and mid-twentieth century German philosopher and psychiatrist Karl Jaspers helped to delineate the irreducible need for meaningful psychological explanation in a psychiatry that was increasingly rooted in causal, neuroscientific explanation. In his great textbook of psychiatry titled *General Psychopathology,* which he published in 1913, Jaspers distinguished between the meaningful approach (*Verstehen*) and the causal approach (*Erklärung*) in clinical psychiatry, and argued for the essential role of both approaches to patient care. Unlike many biological psychiatrists in his day, he believed that psychological meaning could not be eliminated simply because the neurological mechanisms underlying a disease state had been identified. He argued, for example, that the content of a delusional belief is often psychologically meaningful even though the form of the psychopathology (i.e., the delusion itself) is caused by an identifiable disturbance in brain function. Jaspers, in other words, distinguished two aspects of delusions: their presence, which is caused by abnormal brain physiology, and their content, which is explicable only in terms of the individual's psychological dynamics. Jaspers posited that the causal/neuroscientific approach (*Erklärung*) and the meaningful/psychological approach (*Verstehen*) are separate but equally important modes of explanation in psychiatry.

While we are indebted to Jaspers for defining a central role for meaningful psychology in biological psychiatry, his methodological distinction between *Erklärung* and *Verstehen* may be misleading and place unnecessary limitations on psychological explanation. Hundert's analysis of Tim's case suggests why this is the case. Although Jaspers would not have entertained the possibility that Tim's delusion was caused by a meaningful psychological state (such as an unconscious wish or fantasy), Hundert suggested that careful and longitudinal examination of the case revealed such a limitation on causal explanation to be unwarranted. Once Tim had elaborated his delusion, Hundert explained, he felt that he had discovered a compelling reason to go on living: if he took his own life, the world would lose its final opportunity to force Hitler into a personal hell, so that he might suffer for his crimes against humanity. Hundert (1992, 348) stated that Tim's delusion was "an organizing feature of his continued existence," caused in part by meaningful mental states such as the unconscious wish not to commit suicide and the belief that being the reincarnation of Hitler would give him a reason to remain alive. Conversely, the Hitler delusion also can be thought of as causing a reduction in his suicidality. This clinical formulation does not exclude the causal relevance of Tim's well-characterized brain lesions, which might have degraded his capacity to adapt to his condition in an effective and reality-based manner. Instead, the delusion could have been caused by his neurological disease and mental states acting together.

Tim's case is not just of academic interest: it raises important pragmatic, therapeutic questions as well. If Tim's Hitler delusion was caused only by brain dysfunction, then treating that dysfunction directly (perhaps with antipsychotic medications and steroids) would have been clinically necessary and sufficient. But if the delusion was caused in part by mental processes, then treating him with medication alone (while ignoring the causal effects of his psychological motives) might have increased his suicide risk by stripping him of the only part of himself that he considered valuable. Psychotherapy to deal with the painful cognitions and affects that might have contributed to causing the delusion would be necessary in that case as well. Unless Tim came to feel that he had attained emotional security, meaning, and purpose in his life, stripping him of the delusion about Hitler might have been heavy-handed and therapeutically misguided.

For diagnostic and therapeutic reasons, Hundert heeded the psychological factors that seemed to have caused Tim's delusion because failing to do so could have heightened Tim's suffering by depriving him of his raison d'être and thereby increasing his risk for suicide. Even as he applied principles of empirical science to his formulation of Tim's Hitler delusion, Hundert retained an open-minded and longitudinal view of the role of meaningful connections in Tim's life experience. The idea that meaningful states participate in symptom causation may be essential for pragmatic patient care in such cases. Working closely with Tim in long-term psychotherapy, Hundert avoided a restrictive, biological reductionism in which unnecessary limitations are placed on clinical explanation. Meanwhile, by taking available scientific evidence seriously, he did not succumb to an inadequately rigorous eclecticism, in which virtually any concept could count as a valid causal factor. Assuming a pragmatic stance, Hundert strived to work together with Tim in a respectful, scientifically informed, and open-ended manner, all the while acknowledging both the causes of and the rationale for the Hitler delusion—and over time attempting to carefully replace that delusion with a more adaptive and reality-oriented set of thoughts and aspirations.

The idea that meaningful mental states participate in symptom causation may be essential for pragmatic patient care in such cases. To provide patients like Ms. A, Cara, and Tim with effective diagnosis and treatment, psychiatrists should not allow neuroscientific reasoning to cloud their view of people's capacity to experience and to express meaningful mental states. Clinical work with patients like these can be enhanced if psychiatrists employ neuroscientific reasoning in an evidence-based fashion but remain open to the complex and dynamic meanings of human experience and behavior, and to the possibility of changes in that behavior that they could not have predicted. The fact that psychological explanation can be so useful in situations where the relevance of brain-based causal explanation is so undeniable suggests that the ambitious project to merge neurology and psychiatry is seriously flawed. Psychiatrists must vigorously defend, advocate, and teach the humanistic foundations of the discipline in order to prevent neuroscience from becoming its sole foundation.

Neuroscience is one foundation on which clinical psychiatry stands. But so too are the social sciences, humanities, psychology, and other liberal arts that address a broad range of existential and interpersonal concerns in human life. Since clinical psychiatry embraces all these disciplines as equally foundational to its purposes, it must interact closely with clinical neurology but never lose its own identity or sacrifice its humanistic values through an unwarranted merger with neurology grounded in neuroscience alone. As psychiatrists struggle to retain and enhance the unique identity of their field and thereby avoid a reductionistic and antipragmatic merger with neurology, they cannot avoid thinking carefully about the complex nature of their diagnostic system. Will psychiatric diagnoses move toward a pure description of symptoms and avoid any serious consideration of the multidimensional causes (neuroscientific and otherwise) of mental disorders? Or can psychiatry's diagnostic system embrace multiple descriptive and etiological concepts without sacrificing scientific rigor? The abiding challenge of avoiding neurological reductionism and ensuring conceptual pluralism in psychiatric diagnosis is explored in the next chapter.

7

Pragmatism in Psychiatric Diagnosis

The arguments presented so far have critical implications for psychiatric diagnosis, the main focus of this chapter. Cases presented in previous chapters illustrated that clinical pragmatism presupposes a liberal and pluralistic—yet scientifically informed and evidence-based—understanding of what constitutes a causal explanation in the human science of psychiatry. The standard diagnostic system in psychiatry, unfortunately, has not yet embraced this important principle and ought to be updated in the coming years to achieve greater usefulness in clinical settings. This chapter will trace the movement over the last few decades from a relatively nonscientific diagnostic system (which focused on unverified psychodynamic concepts) to the biologically reductive system that we have today, and then go on to suggest how psychiatrists could apply pragmatic principles and causal reasoning to resolve this tension and fine-tune the diagnostic system in the future. In addition, it will delineate a pragmatic approach to the relations among some of the most important diagnostic entities in contemporary and historical psychiatry, including the melancholia of the past and the major depression and "masked depression" of today.

The introduction in 1980 of the third edition of the American Psychiatric Association's *Diagnostic and Statistical Manual of Mental Disorders* (DSM) was a watershed in psychiatry. The first two editions of the manual—DSM-I (1952) and DSM-II (1968)—attempted not only to describe the symptoms of various mental disorders but also to define their etiologies, which were presumed to be psychological. In DSM-I, which was rooted in the psychobiological theory of psychiatrist Adolf Meyer, most mental disorders were understood as "reactions" to stress induced by psychological and interpersonal factors in the person's life. Similarly, in DSM-II, most mental disorders were understood as attempts by the patient to control, ward off, or defend against overwhelming anxiety associated with unconscious, intrapsychic conflicts. The term *neurotic* in DSM-II referred to mental disorders (such as neurotic depression) that were caused in this way. Somatic concepts were employed in DSM-I and DSM-II to specify the cause (and thereby to diagnose) other mental disorders, such as delirium associated with brain dysfunction. A clear division was drawn in the early versions of the DSM between the "organic" mental disorders, which were presumed to be caused by brain pathology, and the "functional disorders," which were thought to be psychogenic (Sullivan 1990).

But with mounting evidence that the "functional" disorders (such as major depression and schizophrenia) were also associated with brain dysfunction and could be treated with psychotropic medications, and with growing skepticism about psychoanalytic explanation in general, a heated debate on the causation and appropriate diagnostic classification of mental disorders was inevitable. By the mid-1970s, there was vehement debate among psychiatrists about whether DSM-II ought to be revised to exclude etiological concepts such as intrapsychic conflict and neurosis. A history of this controversy published by psychiatrists Ronald Bayer and Robert Spitzer (1985)—the latter a major proponent of excluding mental causes from DSM-III diagnostic criteria—described a profession that was divided against itself. On one side were psychotherapists who argued that vast clinical experience had established the validity of a diagnostic approach that employed etiological concepts rooted in psychoanalytic theory. Opposing them were many psychiatrists who believed there was insufficient evidence to justify the claim that the major mental disorders were caused primarily by psychological factors. The latter group championed a more reliable, criteria-based classificatory system that would be silent with regard to the causation of mental disorders but would lend itself well to hypothesis formation and empirical testing.

The later versions of the manual, beginning in 1980 with the DSM-III, represented a particular response to this conflict. DSM-III (1980), its revision DSM-III-R (1987), DSM-IV (1994), and the text revision DSM-IV-TR-(2000) were touted as "atheoretical" classificatory schemes that aimed to specify objective criteria for diagnosing psychiatric disorders, but claimed to state nothing about the causes of those disorders. The transition from mental causation in DSM-II to atheoretical description in the subsequent DSMs was widely deemed a major advance because it empowered researchers and clinicians to speak a common language about mental disorders (a language based on observable symptoms) and to search for more effective treatments of those disorders. Psychiatrists were no longer wedded to a controversial and reductive psychoanalytic model that presumed intrapsychic causation without adequate empirical evidence. After heated debate, the term *neurosis*, which suggested intrapsychic causation, was essentially removed from the new system. The basis for this decision was, in part, the presentation of empirical data that suggested that "neurotic depression" meant different things to different clinicians and therefore could not be diagnosed reliably and consistently (Klerman et al. 1979).

With the introduction of DSM-III, mainstream American psychiatry asserted that its diagnostic system would be based on empirical obser- vation and atheoretical description of mental disorders rather than on certain questionable assumptions about underlying psychological mechanisms and causes of those disorders, as was the case in the previ- ous versions of the manual. DSM-III and each of its successors employed a "multiaxial" diagnostic scheme: Axis I includes the major categories of psychiatric illness, Axis II includes personality disorders and mental retardation, Axis III lists any concomitant medical disorders, Axis IV enumerates any psychosocial stressors affecting the patient's life (such as family problems, poverty, and unemployment), and Axis V specifies a number (on a 0–100 scale) that assesses the patient's global functioning. Whereas DSM-I and DSM-II suggested that psychological factors could cause some mental disorders, DSM-III and the future DSMs specified a multiplicity of factors associated with the disorder (ranging from the medical on Axis III to the psychosocial on Axis IV) but aimed to be silent as to whether those factors actually caused the disorders that appeared on Axes I and II.

Contentious debate continued after 1980 on the relationship between etiological concepts and psychiatric diagnosis. In a highly touted debate on DSM-III published in the *American Journal of Psychiatry* in 1984, two proponents of DSM-III (Spitzer and Gerald Klerman) and two opponents of the new edition of the manual (Robert Michels and George Vaillant) exchanged ideas about the relationship of etiology and description in psychiatric diagnosis (Klerman et al. 1984). On the one hand, Michels and Vaillant both argued that psychiatric diagnosis ignores the issue of causality only at its peril. Noting that DSM-III had abandoned a long-standing notion of intrapsychic dynamics as the etiological basis of most psychiatric illness, Michels bemoaned the fact that "we seem to be veering away from notions of psychologic determinants of those illnesses—a most unusual way of thinking for most psychiatrists" (in Klerman et al. 1984, 549). On the other hand, Klerman and Spitzer defended the effort to delineate categories of mental disorders without making the theoretical commitments that necessarily come along with specifying their causes. Klerman conceded that an ideal diagnostic system would attend to etiology, but argued that psychiatry had not yet advanced to the point where that was possible. "This reliance on descriptive rather than etiologic criteria does not represent an abandonment of the ideal of modern scientific medicine that classification and diagnosis should be by causation," he wrote. "Rather it represents a strategic mode of dealing with the frustrating reality that, for most of the disorders we currently treat, there is only limited evidence for their etiologies" (in Klerman et al. 1984, 540). Considering that the causes of most mental disorders were unknown, it seemed prudent to avoid making causal assumptions in the diagnostic criteria in the DSM.

But despite efforts to achieve a purely atheoretical description of psychiatric diagnostic criteria, the current system does not successfully avoid falling into the trap of making reductive causal assumptions. It turns out to be a myth that DSM-III, DSM-III-R, DSM-IV, and DSM-IV-TR are truly atheoretical in nature. What actually occurred in the decisive transition from DSM-II to DSM-III was that psychological (as well as social) causation essentially was eliminated and replaced in many cases by explicit or implicit biological causation. The debate over whether mental states can play a causal role has taken a decidedly biological and reductive turn in recent years. The case of major mood disorders is a prime example of this phenomenon. DSM-IV empowered clinicians to diagnose "major depressive disorder due to a general medical condition," but not to diagnose "major depressive disorder due to a stressful life event" (p. 366). The same holds true for bipolar disorder and a host of other conditions, such as anxiety disorders and psychotic disorders. Along these lines, William Follette and Arthur Houts (1996, 1120) noted that "the modern DSMs may avoid explicating their theoretical underpinnings, but the underlying ontologies of a weakly stated medical model are easily deducible from their content." This consideration suggests a disturbing twofold inconsistency in the diagnostic system.

In the first place, the fact that DSM-IV still allows mood disorders like major depression to be "due to" anything at all suggests that the diagnostic system is not in fact atheoretical, as its proponents have claimed. Instead, the theory implied by this approach is that biological factors, in the form of general medical conditions and substance abuse disorders, are causally powerful and therefore are relevant to making diagnoses in psychiatry, whereas psychosocial factors are not. This theoretical commitment has become more solidified with the progression from DSM-III to DSM-IV. Spitzer and other early framers of the DSM-III led a movement in the early 1990s to retire the term *organic* from the DSM-III-R and to replace it with the phrases "substance-induced" or "due to a general medical condition" in the DSM-IV (Spitzer et al. 1992). They argued that the traditional organic/functional dichotomy in psychiatry was problematic, because it implied that some mental disorders were due to psychological factors and thus it was "at variance with the growing body of evidence of the importance of biological factors in the etiology of the major 'nonorganic' mental disorders" (p. 241). Excluding the familiar term *organic* from the DSM-IV implied, ironically, that all disorders were organic. Far from being atheoretical, DSM-IV suggested that some mood disorders result from substances or general medical conditions, but not from psychosocial factors. Eliminating the organic/functional dichotomy from the manual ensured against any confusion regarding this distinctly theoretical stance in the DSM-IV.

In the second place, assuming that it is indeed acceptable to acknowledge causation in the DSM, it seems prejudicial to grant general medical or substance-induced conditions a prominent place in the diagnostic scheme without doing the same for psychosocial events. Numerous empirical studies have suggested that stressful life events can cause major depressive episodes (Kendler, Karkowski, and Prescott 1999; Paykel 1978). But, unfortunately, DSM-IV does not acknowledge mood disorder due to a stressful life event as a category of illness on Axis I, where the major diagnoses are listed. Meanwhile, Axis IV, where the psychosocial stressors in a particular case are enumerated, is silent with respect to the causation of mental disorders. Spitzer and his colleagues (1992, 243) have advocated prejudicially for the retention on Axis I of causal qualifiers for general medical and substance-induced factors, but not for psychosocial factors: they asserted that "the clinical judgment about the etiologic role of 'organic' factors is often extremely difficult and sometimes impossible, but eliminating this treatment-relevant distinction from our nosology hardly seems to represent an advance." But they failed to make the equally cogent point that, while it is difficult to know if and how a psychosocial event contributed to causation of a mental disorder, eliminating notation of that event from Axis I and consigning it to Axis IV may have negative consequences for treatment planning. The exclusion of psychological and social causes from Axis I is ad hoc, prejudicial, and reductive.

There is no principled reason for excluding mental causes from Axis I, however. In fact, DSM-IV already acknowledges psychosocial causation of major psychiatric illness in some limited cases, such as in posttraumatic stress disorder (PTSD), which is conceived of as the result of a traumatic event and a subjective response that is characterized by "intense fear, helplessness, or horror" (p. 428). In addition, DSM-IV understands conversion disorder primarily as the result of unconscious intrapsychic conflicts; the manual states that in conversion disorder, "psychological factors are judged to be associated with the symptom or deficit because the initiation or exacerbation of the symptom or deficit is preceded by conflicts or other stressors" (p. 457). Malingering and factitious disorder are two other examples of Axis I diagnoses with presumed psychological causes. They differ from conversion disorder insofar as the psychological cause of the presenting symptom or deficit is conscious and intentional. While the motive for symptom production in malingering is an external incentive, the motive for abnormal behavior in factitious disorder is assumption of the sick role. In both cases, however, DSM-IV acknowledges that symptoms are caused by psychological factors. But

PTSD, conversion disorder, factitious disorder, and malingering are exceptions to the rule in DSM-IV, which asserts that many major Axis I disorders may be caused by substance abuse or by a general medical condition, but not by a psychosocial factor. Such constriction of psychosocial causation flies in the face of empirical research findings and widely held philosophical assumptions about human behavior.

These considerations lead to two possible proposals for improving the DSM in the future. One possibility, already suggested by Barry Fogel (1990), would be to make the DSM purely descriptive by removing all suggestions of causation of mental disorders, including the labels "substance-induced" and "due to a general medical condition" on Axis I. General medical conditions, such as complex partial seizures and hypothyroidism, would continue to appear on Axis III, as they do under the current system, but they would no longer appear on Axis I as causal explanations of the major psychiatric disorders. Likewise, a list of psychosocial stressors would continue to appear on Axis IV, but never on Axis I. This approach would render the DSM more descriptive and atheoretical than it is currently because neither biological nor psychosocial causes would be considered for the purpose of diagnosis. At the same time, however, exercising this option would be problematic and impractical, because it would limit the clinician's capacity to incorporate into psychiatric diagnoses some highly relevant and valid etiological data. Excluding etiological data from major Axis I diagnoses in turn could have a detrimental effect on treatment planning, because failing to specify the presumed causes of mental disorders may impoverish the therapeutic approach that the clinician could bring to bear.

A pragmatic alternative would be to make the diagnostic system more flexible and pluralistic by permitting careful reintroduction in certain instances of psychosocial causes on Axis I. Clearly, many major diagnoses that are caused by biomedical factors alone, such as delirium, would not be affected by liberalizing the use of psychosocial causes on Axis I. But the fact that some Axis I disorders have no clear psychosocial cause does not imply that others do not. In the case of a patient with bipolar disorder who becomes depressed following a death of a family member and failure to adhere to the prescribed medication regimen, the Axis I diagnosis might be "bipolar disorder, current episode depressed due to a stressful life event and medication noncompliance." One could envision in a future DSM other pluralistic psychiatric diagnoses, such as "major depressive episode due to a genetic vulnerability, a thyroid illness, and a stressful life event." As we have seen, there is as much empirical evidence that stressful life events can cause major depressive episodes as there is that genetic, metabolic, or substance-related factors can do so. There is no compelling reason why future DSMs should not be receptive to the possibility that a wide array of factors, ranging from the biological to the psychosocial, contribute to the onset of Axis I mood disorders, in accordance with the pluralistic approach suggested by clinical pragmatism.

There are likely to be many good ways to operationalize this idea in future versions of the DSM. While it is unnecessary at this point to specify just one way of incorporating psychosocial causation into Axis I mood disorder diagnoses, a possible solution is as follows. First of all, it would be imprudent to make abrupt and major changes in the current diagnostic criteria, because they already have gained widespread consensual agreement and are the basis of a great deal of research. But it might be reasonable to start by removing the diagnoses "major depressive disorder due to a general medical condition" and "substance-induced major depressive disorder," but retain the diagnosis "major depressive disorder." This would satisfy the scientific impulse toward purely descriptive and atheoretical diagnosis on Axis I. However, within the diagnostic criteria for major depressive disorder, a future DSM could allow clinicians to specify one or more causes of an episode of major depression, including (but not limited to) medical conditions, substance-induced conditions, and psychosocial factors—as long as there was plausible empirical evidence suggesting such causality. This would satisfy the impulse to acknowledge the reality of multifactorial causation and would lead psychiatrists to more pragmatic, multidimensional, and interdisciplinary treatment planning. Since specification of various causal factors could evolve and deepen as clinician and patient get to know each other better over a long period of time, the core pragmatic values of methodological pluralism, participatory and collaborative care, and provisional explanation would be fully incorporated into the diagnostic process.

This second proposal for improving the DSM in the future is much more exciting and timely than the first, because it would help to enhance treatment planning and promote conceptual integration of the field. A pluralistic diagnostic system could improve treatment planning substantially by reminding clinicians about the importance of psychosocial interventions for many Axis I disorders, including mood disorders. By confidently asserting that major Axis I disorders can result from psychosocial factors, a new and improved DSM might help to convince insurance companies and managed-care organizations that paying for a wide variety of psychosocial treatments—not just medication management—is ethical and cost-effective. Acceptance of multifactorial causation in psychiatric diagnosis would cohere with philosopher Hilary Putnam's suggestion (1999) that explanations of human behavior always should subsume "a plurality of conceptual resources." It would help us approach psychiatrist Leon Eisenberg's (1986) compelling vision of a clinical psychiatry that is neither "brainless" nor "mindless." As psychiatrists consider what changes in DSM-IV would lead to creation of a more theoretically sound and pragmatically oriented DSM-V, they should work toward making multifactorial causation and provisional case formulation as much a part of formal diagnosis as they are of everyday practice. The complexity of the conditions with which patients suffer demands no less.

Reformulating psychiatric diagnoses to adhere to the four *p*'s of clinical pragmatism will be an exercise in defining ethical values as much as it will be about refining psychiatric science. Psychiatrist John Sadler for many years has argued cogently that considerations of value are just as important as considerations of scientific fact in the development of a sound diagnostic system (Sadler 1997, 2002, 2004; also Sadler, Hulgusa, and Agich 1994). Sadler has drawn a telling analogy that highlights the status of psychiatric diagnoses in everyday practice. A gardener clearly needs to know a great deal about flowers and plants to achieve the desired aesthetic effects, but it is not necessary to know every scientific detail about the proper categorization of plants that the academic botanist has mastered. The gardener and the botanist have distinct (though compatible) ways of categorizing flowers and plants. Neither approach is more valid than the other—each is valid only inasmuch as it serves the gardener's or the botanist's respective practical goals.

The same goes for psychiatric diagnoses. Geneticists may eventually be able to divide patients into distinct categories—such as those with mild, moderate, or severe vulnerabilities to major depression—based on empirical scientific tests. There are already promising laboratory tests that may be able to divide patients into such categories based on variations in their genetic blueprints for a protein that is responsible for how the brain handles the neurotransmitter serotonin, which is a major biochemical factor in depression and is affected by serotonin reuptake inhibitor medications such as Prozac. Clinical psychiatrists will need to be aware of these genetically based categories as they assess patients and consider various treatment options. But to develop appropriate treatment plans for their individual patients, they may use a different system of categorization that is based on other practical factors, such as patients' willingness to take psychotropic medications and/or engage in psychotherapy. Diagnosing a patient with a genetic anomaly may lead to effective treatment with psychotropic medication, but if the patient is unwilling to take the medication (Ms. A's situation as described in chapter 6), the psychiatrist will need other intelligible ways to locate the patient and to offer something helpful (psychodynamic therapy in Ms. A's case). Diagnosis in these cases is guided by the uniqueness of individual patients rather than by the generalizations of empirical science. Psychologist Peter Zachar (2000, 2003) argued that diagnostic categories in psychiatry are not "natural kinds," which he defined as bounded and objective categories that "carve nature at the joints," but instead are "practical kinds," which are flexible and pragmatic categorizations that help psychiatrists navigate the everyday clinical world and help patients achieve their goals.

How might pragmatic values be used to define specific diagnostic entities in clinical psychiatry? Among the most prevalent and crippling disorders that can be considered from the standpoint of pragmatic values and that can be regarded as practical kinds are the mood disorders, which have been conceptualized in many different ways over the course of the centuries. The melancholia of the past and the major depression of the present day are extraordinarily complex notions that represent different things to different people. In an article titled "Is This Dame Melancholy? Equating Today's Depression and Past Melancholia," philosopher Jennifer Radden (2003) made an important contribution to the debate on whether these diagnostic concepts should be seen as identical, overlapping, or distinct categories. Exploring both conditions from the descriptive and the causal points of view, Radden concluded that fully equating them would constitute a "troubling oversimplification." Because past descriptions of melancholia and current descriptions of major depression are marked by dissimilarities (e.g., the genius and creativity that are associated with the former and the self-loathing and emphasis on loss that are associated with the latter), only an underlying causal base common to both conditions would justify equating them. But the cause (or causes) of melancholia and major depression remain mysterious. Thus, although Radden acknowledged that a causal explanation might yield substantial benefits ("research possibilities, further hypotheses, and even hope of prevention, or cure"), she suggested that we remain in a descriptive mode when comparing the two conditions and therefore concluded that they are not one and the same.

Radden's argument that past melancholia and contemporary depression are descriptively distinct is convincing and indisputable. But while Radden is correct that the cause of many (or perhaps most) depressive states is unknown, she underrates the extent of the empirical knowledge that we have acquired about the causation of depression and, in so doing, undervalues the relevance of causal reasoning to making the melancholia/depression distinction. Recent empirical research has revealed that major depressive episodes can result from brain lesions such as left-sided strokes or from metabolic disorders such as hypothyroidism. Psychosocial research, moreover, has suggested that stressful life events can be understood as causes of depression. These findings provide some hope that the identification of causes of various clinical states is a real possibility. Identification of such causes could empower psychiatrists to make some plausible claims about the similarities or differences between past melancholia and current depression. A melancholic individual like the artist Vincent van Gogh, for example, had a different illness than a contemporary stroke patient with depression in a present-day hospital not only on the basis of the descriptive distinctions between their conditions, but also on the basis of the causes of their respective states. Although we cannot know the cause of Van Gogh's melancholia, we can assume that it was not the result of a left-sided stroke due to the absence in his case of other clinical deficits that often result from such a stroke, such as right-sided weakness and language deficits. Plausible assertions about the causation of melancholic and depressive states would add to the legitimacy of claims regarding the distinctness of the conditions.

Conversely, careful consideration of the etiology of various clinical presentations might prompt us to hypothesize a shared pathophysiology and thereby lead us to believe that they are essentially identical conditions. It is difficult or impossible to discover a cause of melancholia in individuals who lived in past eras. But we might achieve this goal by comparing well-defined major depression to various forms of "masked depression," such as those seen in cross-cultural settings, where the subjective symptoms of sad mood are absent but many somatic signs of depression (such as anorexia, slowness of bodily movement, and cognitive deficits) are observed. If it turned out that major depression and "masked depression" had the same underlying cause, then differences in their clinical phenomenology would be merely surface differences that belie a shared etiological process.

How might one discover the existence of such a process? One method would involve the "drug cartography" that Radden discussed but essentially dismissed in her article. Drug cartography involves establishment of diagnostic categories on the basis of common responses of various symptoms to the very same pharmacological treatment. Based on the favorable response to certain antidepressant medications of eight distinct medical/psychiatric conditions (major depression, bulimia nervosa, panic disorder, obsessive-compulsive disorder, attention deficit disorder with hyperactivity, cataplexy, migraine, and irritable bowel syndrome), psychiatrists James Hudson and Harrison Pope (1990) have argued that these disorders may share a common pathophysiological abnormality and thus could be understood as a single disorder, which they refer to as "affective spectrum disorder." Although their hypothesis is unproven, its plausibility and testability suggest the relevance of causal reasoning to the development of novel hypotheses about the relations among various conditions in medicine and psychiatry. Cellular, genetic, or neuroimaging research might prove or disprove the theory of affective spectrum disorder. But if psychiatrists were to adhere strictly to Radden's call for the adoption of "descriptivism" in psychiatric diagnosis, such a research program might never get off the ground.

This would be a shame not only for theoretical but also for practical reasons. Radden mentioned (but did not pursue in depth) the possible role of pragmatic reasoning in conceiving the relations among past melancholia and contemporary depression and masked depression. In fact, she stated explicitly that an ontological approach to the causal/descriptive debate over these relationships is preferable to any approach that is "merely pragmatic." But, unfortunately, she did not explain or justify her rationale for adopting this particular theoretical orientation. Pragmatic considerations ought to be foremost as philosophers and psychiatrists grapple with the complexities of psychiatric explanation. They should also be prominent when considering the complicated questions that Radden raised and adroitly defined. From the researcher's standpoint, successful investigation of the differences among melancholia, major depression, and masked depression may depend more on the development of hypotheses about underlying causes than on further observations of symptomatic differences among them. Moreover, from the clinician's standpoint, the ultimate goal of exploring these questions in the first place is to fine-tune their diagnostic and therapeutic methodologies for the sake of enhancing patient care.

In this debate over the relationships among melancholia and depression and masked depression, then, we must ask what is at stake for the real-world patients who present to psychiatrists' offices seeking relief from their suffering. Deliberations about whether these conditions are identical or distinct cannot be divorced from considerations of the practical effects of these deliberations on the clinical care individuals receive. Open-minded assessment of the causation of depressive disorders can have practical benefits for diagnosis, for research (e.g., on affective spectrum disorder), and for treatment (e.g., of correctable metabolic disorders, such as hypothyroidism). In addition, acknowledgment of a plurality of causal factors in psychiatry's main diagnostic system might help psychiatrists make a strong case to third-party payers that reimbursing for pluralistic evaluation and treatment planning is scientifically grounded, ethical, and cost-effective.

Although in her article Radden chose not to focus on the pragmatic dimensions of the philosophical debate she addressed, her conclusion that past melancholia and current depression are distinct nevertheless has some pragmatic implications for contemporary psychiatry. One of the most important corollaries of Radden's arguments lies in its subtle and sophisticated reminder to clinicians that the person experiencing subjective sadness or melancholia cannot be reduced to (or equated with) observable, "neurovegetative" signs of major depression. The depressed person in our own times, we must presume, has an inner world that is as rich and complex as that of the melancholic person of the past. The meaningful dimensions of personal experience shape the nature and course of mental disorder as much as the causal dimensions. If clinicians do not recognize the subjectively "melancholic" person who is living behind the objectively "depressed" clinical presentation, they might fail to diagnose and treat the person in an empathic and individualized way. For example, they might resort to completion of symptom checklists and rating scales rather than commit their time and energy to the development of an individually tailored clinical formulation and treatment plan.

Sadly, this form of psychiatric evaluation has expanded in recent years with worsening financial constraints on our health-care systems. The resulting neglect of distinctions between the subjective experiences and objective signs of depression—and the reduction of the former to the latter—has placed unfortunate limitations on treatment options and also threatens the scope of clinical research. Radden's emphasis on the complicated subjective natures of melancholia and depression, her rigorous consideration of the causal and descriptive dimensions of both states, and her insistence on respecting the diagnostic differences between them serve as a much-needed antidote to this impoverishing trend. Fighting this trend is a matter of scientific concern as psychiatrists work on reforming the DSM and strive to diagnose and treat patients in an individualized but evidence-based fashion.

It is also a matter of human values. The contemporary diagnostic system in psychiatry values the biomedical approach over the psychological approach to many disorders, such as depression. At a time when we are still struggling with a rather elementary understanding of most mental disorders, the diagnostic system reflects more about psychiatric ethics than it does about psychiatric science. Will the prejudicial tendency to allow biomedical causes, but not psychosocial causes, to appear on Axis I continue in the future DSMs, and thereby support treatment approaches that favor medications over psychotherapy? Or will psychiatrists in the future choose to value the practical, pluralistic, participatory, and provisional dimensions of clinical explanation and diagnosis—and thereby keep multiple treatment options in play? Can philosophical pragmatism ground psychiatric ethics and guide clinical practice in the twenty-first century? What kinds of educational and research programs would need to be in place to promote the four *p*'s in clinical psychiatry? What, I ask in the eighth and final chapter, is the future of psychiatry and how might it embrace the major principles of clinical pragmatism in the years ahead?

8

Pragmatism and the Future of Psychiatry

The disorder in twenty-first-century psychiatry is all about the search to integrate human values. The practicing psychiatrist today is constantly trying to negotiate compelling pulls toward the values of science and the values of humanism. In a postmodern era, with no objective moral or conceptual compass to orient today's practitioner, the world of clinical psychiatry remains messy and ill-defined. Clinicians at times may be tempted to adopt the values of scientific reductionism, which trades an appreciation of human complexity and subjectivity for the order and certainty of coherent systems and testable theories. At other times they may be tempted to adopt the values of humanism, which acknowledges the complexity of the human drama but does so only at the expense of sacrificing the conceptual benefits of a well-ordered, evidence-based approach to diagnosis, formulation, and treatment. With ongoing advances in psychiatric science, the impulse toward reductionism likely will intensify. But with inherent limitations on scientific reasoning as applied to complex and unpredictable human behavior, the principles of humanism cannot be wished away or explained away. How will the twenty-first-century psychiatrist negotiate the competing values of science and humanism?

The key challenge in this setting is to balance these competing values by identifying a set of values that are compatible with, but can also transcend, pure science or pure humanism. This challenge, in essence, is not an empirical one. Burgeoning knowledge in psychiatric science—even Churchland's notion of a "completed neuroscience"—would never be able to heal the disorder of values in clinical psychiatry. Questions about whether and how to apply that science, and concerns about preserving the dignity and decision-making authority of the individual patient, are merely a couple of the many factors that will keep considerations of ethical values at the forefront of psychiatric thinking in the twenty-first century. Similarly, the challenge is not abstract or philosophical in nature: psychiatrists cannot simply think their way to an acceptable solution to the science/humanism problem. Instead, the challenge that psychiatrists face is an ethical one at its core: only by defining the central values of their field can psychiatrists figure out how to explain the emotional suffering they witness each day, to place the persons they treat into workable categories of disease and suffering, and to apply the emerging brain and behavioral sciences sensibly and compassionately.

Clinical pragmatism, rooted in a distinctively American philosophy of the nineteenth and twentieth centuries, provides a theoretical foundation from which a whole system of psychiatric ethics in the twenty-first century can arise. It is not burdened by the shortcomings of scientific and philosophical systems of thought (such as consilience and eliminative materialism) that dictate absolutely correct or incorrect forms of reasoning. On the contrary, clinical pragmatism aims humbly to develop a workable map that depicts how psychiatry ought to move in the future and how it can use all of its foundational sciences—ranging from the neurosciences to psychology and the liberal arts—in a thoughtful and coherent manner. Its core ethical value is the primacy of practical results for individual persons in the everyday life world. Scientific data and philosophical systems do not have primacy for the pragmatic psychiatrist, though they often play useful roles in helping individual patients achieve the practical results they desire. Clinical pragmatism suggests a method for defining what a favorable practical result looks like: it does not define a good result from an abstract or objective vantage point, but rather in terms of the deliberations and negotiations among the people working toward those goals. It is not static but remains open to changes in every conceivable domain, including changes in empirical data based on new research studies and changes in people's goals as their lives evolve in the face of new circumstances and challenges.

The pragmatic psychiatrist considers it unethical to privilege theory over practical results, to place limits on the use of concepts and methods that may help to achieve those results, to make heavy-handed decisions without the participation of the patient, and to see greater certainty in clinical situations than really exists at any given time. By guiding practice in accordance with the four *p*'s, clinical pragmatism opens up a fresh new approach to psychiatric ethics in the twenty-first century. Applying the four *p*'s of clinical pragmatism in everyday practice helps define a fifth *p* that can guide psychiatric ethics in the future: professionalism. In keeping with the roots of the term *professionalism* in the age-old notion of professing a vow of service to others, the pragmatic psychiatrist makes an ethical commitment to basing all clinical work on the values of practical outcomes, pluralistic explanatory tools and treatment interventions, participation of patients as collaborators, and provisional and humble sensibilities about all aspects of the work. The professionalism of the pragmatic psychiatrist is a form of the "mindful practice" defined by physician Ronald Epstein (1999, 833) as the use of "critical self-reflection" that enables the clinician to "listen attentively to patients' distress, recognize their own errors, refine their technical skills, make evidence-based decisions, and clarify their values so that they can act with compassion, technical competence, presence, and insight."

So what will psychiatric ethics in the twenty-first century look like? In recent years, psychiatric ethics has focused on many challenges to the doctor-patient relationship. The third edition of the comprehensive volume *Psychiatric Ethics* (Bloch, Chodoff, and Green 1999) provides clear evidence of the widening scope of the field. Included in the volume are chapters on the ethical aspects of confidentiality, involuntary treatment, managed care, health resource allocation, clinical research, and psychiatric education. Each of these chapters defines an essential aspect of sound practice in psychiatry. But recently psychiatric ethicists have also focused on explaining psychiatric disorders, negotiating the dialectic of science and humanism, and clarifying the complex relation between reductive and eclectic approaches to diagnosis, case formulation, and treatment. In a chapter of *Psychiatric Ethics* titled "Analytic Philosophy, Brain Science, and the Concept of Disorder," philosopher K.W.M. Fulford (1999) argued that ethical considerations ought to be just as much at the core of psychiatry's explanatory models as are scientific findings and biomedical reasoning. In the "fact-plus-value model" of psychiatric disorder, according to Fulford, "science and the humanities are equally essential to good clinical care" (p. 187). Fulford aims to promote ethical practice and thereby heal the science/humanism divide in psychiatry by paying serious attention to both sides of the long-standing conceptual and methodological divide in the field.

The expansion of psychiatric ethics to address questions about the values underlying clinical explanations is a much-needed development. Explanations of mental disorders inevitably lead to practical decisions about how to treat them. Conversely, available treatment modalities determine the nature and the content of clinical case formulations. If, for example, psychodynamic psychotherapy were not available in a particular treatment setting (perhaps due to financial limitations imposed by a managed-care organization), a patient's distress would not be conceptualized in terms of transference distortions or problematic object relations. And if medically trained psychiatrists were not diagnosing and treating mental disorders (perhaps because it is less costly to have non-M.D. clinicians perform these tasks), patients might not benefit from advances in neuroscience and psychopharmacology. Explanatory models in psychiatry have ethical significance because they reflect what psychiatrists deem valuable in clinical presentations and they lead clinicians to practical treatment decisions. The pragmatic psychiatrist attends carefully to the values that underlie clinical work because those values guide the diagnostic and treatment methods that ultimately are made available to deliver the optimal treatment to each and every patient.

Appreciating both sides of the science/humanism continuum, psychiatrist Roger Sider (1984, 390) wrote that "psychiatrists usually select therapeutic modalities for their patients on the basis of empirical and theoretical considerations," but he went on to state that "every therapeutic decision involves questions of value and requires ethical justification." This principle has been elaborated in the last decade by psychiatric ethicists such as Fulford, who delineated the ethical imperative of integrating scientific facts and ethical values for the sake of crafting good clinical explanations and effective therapies. In a paper on the place of psychiatric ethics in the larger realm of biomedical ethics, Fulford and Tony Hope (1994, 693) suggested that psychiatrists should adopt a "full-field view" of explanation in which "value is incorporated on an equal basis with fact." Fulford and Hope believe a "fact-plus-value model" of psychiatric care has important implications for practice. It raises the profile of ethics in psychiatry by highlighting that considerations of value could never be displaced by biomedical science, regardless of how far that science may advance. It does not limit the critical role evidence-based biomedicine rightfully will play in the psychiatry of the future, but it instead conceives of science and ethics as equal partners in clinical explanation and treatment. Furthermore, it has profound implications for the organization of health-care services, psychiatric training, and psychiatric research—each of which I will address in this chapter.

The pragmatic psychiatrist is a broadly trained and open-minded patient advocate with a deep ethical commitment to a practical, pluralistic, participatory, provisional, and professional approach to persons in treatment. Every practicing psychiatrist in the twenty-first century ought to strive to implement all the values of clinical pragmatism. But the commitments of the pragmatic psychiatrist may differ at times from those of some psychiatric researchers and highly specialized clinicians, who in their roles focus on scientific aspects of psychiatry in order to elucidate mechanisms of disease or advance knowledge. Psychopharmacologists who conduct clinical trials of psychotropic medications, for example, assume the important task of carefully investigating whether a medication is more efficacious than a placebo for a well-defined set of symptoms in a relatively homogeneous set of patients. Neuroimaging psychiatrists may use technologies, such as functional magnetic resonance imaging (fMRI) or magnetic resonance spectroscopy (MRS), to elucidate which brain regions and chemicals undelie critical mental functions (such as perception, memory, and affect) in persons with and without psychiatric illness. The basic research of psychiatric scientists and the clinical research of psychiatric specialists provide important prospects for improvements of patient care in the years to come.

Meanwhile, the pragmatic psychiatrist draws on this accumulation of scientific knowledge but keeps things in balance for the sake of preserving the patient's best interests in the present. A practical, pluralistic, participatory, provisional, and professional approach empowers the patient and the clinician to make good use of empirical knowledge in a highly contextualized fashion, with an unswerving focus on application of relevant clinical science to the patient's unique situation, characteristics, and personal wishes. The pragmatic psychiatrist must advocate for and make good use of empirical research findings, but at the same time assume a practical and individually tailored stance when applying such findings in particular cases. Pragmatism in clinical psychiatry calls for a primary focus on the individual patient rather than on a particular disease, diagnosis, drug, neurotransmitter, neuroimaging technology, or gene. The pragmatically oriented psychiatrist in the twenty-first century can ensure that scientific knowledge of the human brain and behavior is vigorously pursued even as human values and rights are acknowledged, protected, and enhanced in day-to-day clinical encounters.

Pragmatic psychiatrists can and should promote this line of thinking not only in their own clinical practices, but also in settings that influence general practice. An open-ended and evolving clinical discipline like psychiatry always orients itself to the future. Ensuring the availability of pragmatic psychiatric care in years to come will depend on the nature of educational and research programs implemented today. Luhrmann's anthropological analysis depicted how psychiatrists-in-training are too often indoctrinated into only one of two models of psychiatric explanation and treatment: the biomedical or the psychodynamic. She feared that, with the ongoing growth of clinical neuroscience and the expansion of managed care, the role of expensive, long-term psychotherapy in contemporary psychiatry would continue to wane. If indeed this were to occur, Luhrmann (2000, 24) noted, "There is a possibility that our psychiatrists, and perhaps our society, will learn to see even less complexity than before."

What would result from expanding the trainee's focus on neuroscience but restricting his or her exposure to long-term psychotherapy? The scenario that most concerns Luhrmann and me is one in which the teaching of neuroscience to psychiatric residents becomes so prominent and so highly valued that it excludes the teaching of humanistic approaches to psychiatric explanation and treatment. Restriction of the humanistic approaches in psychiatric training would run counter to the pluralistic values of clinical pragmatism and thereby threaten to narrow the wide range of approaches psychiatric residents need to learn in order to become ethical and effective clinical practitioners. Without a commitment to pluralism in psychiatric education today, there would be a paucity of pragmatic psychiatrists in the future, and patients in the future would be deprived of the multidimensional therapeutic options they desire and deserve. Psychiatrist and former residency training director John Nemiah (1981, 192) argued more than 20 years ago that psychiatric residents need an "educational experience that will enable them to weave together the biological and the psychodynamic into an organic synthesis that is greater than either part alone." His point remains just as relevant today.

To address the concerns that Luhrmann and Nemiah so aptly described, psychiatric educators and residency training directors must assume the challenge of balancing clinical and didactic experiences so the psychiatrist of the future is intellectually equipped to coordinate diverse explanatory concepts and treatment modalities in order to provide ethical and pragmatic patient care. Solid training in neurology will be necessary but not sufficient for achieving this goal. Collapsing psychiatry training into neuroscience training would run the risk of restricting the depth of psychodynamic and psychosocial education of residents, who must learn early in their training the importance of casting a wide conceptual net in diagnosis and treatment. One way to accomplish this teaching goal is to encourage residents to work with patients who need comprehensive care targeted at neuropsychiatric, psychopharmacological, psychotherapeutic, and interpersonal difficulties. Patients with complex clinical problems are ideal for trainees to learn from and to treat because they demonstrate the pluralistic nature of mental illness, the indeterminate and open-ended nature of such illness, and the ethical imperative to provide care that involves the patient as a coparticipant in decision making. They also demonstrate to trainees how important it is to manage uncertainty and to maintain intellectual humility in the face of the overwhelming amounts of knowledge and know-how that clinical psychiatrists must strive to master.

It is critical to help psychiatrists in training to become pragmatically oriented practitioners by ensuring that they are taught and supervised by role models who do not restrict themselves to one camp or school of thought in psychiatry. While it may be necessary for trainees to learn about specialized models from psychiatrists who assume a scientific approach in their areas of interest (such as neuroimaging specialists, psychopharmacologists, and cognitive psychologists), the teachers and supervisors with whom trainees interact most frequently and intensively should model clinical pragmatism by focusing primarily on achieving favorable treatment outcomes, considering multiple aspects of patients' presentations, engaging respectfully and collaboratively with patients, acknowledging limitations, and managing uncertainty. Such supervisors model for psychiatric trainees the principle that one can think about cases in a rigorous and evidence-based fashion without slipping into reductionism. At the same time, they demonstrate that psychiatric clinicians can attend carefully to human variation, complexity, and psychodynamic meaning without sacrificing rigor or slipping into postmodernism. Learning to see people from multiple points of view, and to shift from one point of view to another in a pragmatically guided manner, ought to be at the core of a contemporary psychiatric education. Some trainees will go on to highly specialized careers in particular areas of psychiatry, but a pragmatically oriented clinical education is likely to help them achieve greater breadth, nuance, and sensitivity in their future work as clinicians and/or researchers.

Open-ended, multifactorial explanatory models in psychiatry necessitate the integration of neuropsychiatric, psychopharmacological, psychotherapeutic, and family- and community-oriented treatments. In an era of growing concern for the escalating costs of health care, it may seem problematic that such models would suggest a need for more rather than less treatment availability, and therefore lead to increased rather than decreased expenditures of financial resources. But it is reasonable for psychiatrists to argue that more spending on mental health care is valuable and does not squander precious resources. Indeed, evidence has emerged that comprehensive psychiatric care actually can, in the long run, reduce spending on both general medical care and mental health care (Doidge 1997; Gabbard et al. 1997; Stone 2001). But in addition, while psychiatrists increasingly are being called on to ensure that their work is evidence-based and cost-effective, they need not accept the notion that cutting health-care costs is always desirable. In the end, effective and multimodal care in psychiatry will only come at substantial costs, but costs that psychiatrists can and should demonstrate are worthwhile for individuals, families, workplaces, and communities.

Psychiatrists see in everyday practice that their work is practical, that it enhances people's enjoyment of life and their ability to function at home and at work, and therefore that it is highly valuable to individual patients, families, employers, and society in general. Comprehensive and pragmatic psychiatry—even if expensive in the short run—promotes economic values as much as it promotes basic human values and societal well-being. Both public and private insurance companies have not yet fully understood that paying for excellent mental health care has innumerable long-term benefits. In the meantime, as psychiatrists Stephen Green and Sidney Bloch (2001) argued in "Working in a Flawed Mental Health Care System: An Ethical Challenge," psychiatrists will have to find creative ways to practice ethically even if managed health-care systems and insurance organizations are not designed to provide or to support appropriate psychiatric treatment. Unfortunately, that will sometimes involve the patient's having to pay out-of-pocket fees for comprehensive treatment or the clinician's having to forgo fair payment for providing noncovered services that may be essential to the patient's well-being.

Pragmatic psychiatry in the future will depend not only on the provision of comprehensive clinical services, but also on discovery of new knowledge about human experience and behavior. How will psychiatrists acquire this knowledge while at the same time ensuring that their patients in the future are not unduly exposed to experimental treatment approaches that may not be effective or safe? The need for broad-spectrum clinical and educational approaches in psychiatry reverberates with the need for multidimensional research that looks with care and rigor at the causes and treatments of mental disorders. Pharmaceutical companies spend millions of dollars to develop and test new medications for conditions ranging from anxiety to depression to psychosis. The goal of this research is to study investigational new drugs so they may obtain U.S. Food and Drug Administration (FDA) approval and acceptance in the marketplace, often yielding clinical benefits to patients and monetary benefits to shareholders. The research is supposed to demonstrate that the treatments are not only effective, but also safe and well tolerated.

Despite growing distrust of the FDA's ability to ensure that only safe and effective medications are approved and marketed, it today remains the foremost organization demanding appropriate testing of new medications. How can the FDA and other organizational bodies (such as professional journals and consumer organizations) ensure that published research on psychiatric treatments is not biased? With growing recognition that researchers tend to publish the positive findings of their research studies more often than negative findings, there is now appropriate concern that all relevant information about psychiatric medications may not be readily available. A handful of published studies may suggest that a psychotropic medication is safe and effective, but how are clinicians and patients to know whether contrary data has been withheld from publication because it is unfavorable to the researcher conducting it or to the company paying for it? There is a growing movement in favor of registering clinical trials so that all results of medical research are automatically made available to the public, not just results that would be financially favorable to the pharmaceutical industry (Dickersin and Rennie 2003). Professional journals in the future could choose to publish only those research studies that have been appropriately registered, so that they avoid the danger of publishing only favorable findings for a medication but never even seeing negative findings because researchers and corporate sponsors of research have never submitted them for publication.

Registration of clinical trials is one avenue toward making sweeping changes in how psychiatric research is conducted and reported. But it is equally critical to ensure that research is safe and appropriate for each individual who chooses to participate. How can people who volunteer to participate in clinical trials be protected, and at the same time how can researchers learn something new that might help the individual subject and millions of other people in the future? Like everyday patient care, clinical research in psychiatry ought to be a pragmatic enterprise that resolves the tension between the scientific quest for knowledge and the everyday human needs of individuals. Clinical researchers necessarily strive for empirical knowledge gained by the study of human subjects, but at the same time clinical researchers need to respect the fundamental human rights of each individual subject. The goals of clinical treatment and clinical research diverge: the former aims for pragmatically based care of individual persons, while the latter aims for rigorous scientific data. Nonetheless, the major tenets of clinical pragmatism apply even in the context of clinical research, where the basic aim is to enhance the quality of psychiatric care in the future while protecting the health and welfare of research subjects in the present.

Applying core pragmatic principles to enhance the ethics of psychiatric research programs is a responsibility that members of the institutional review board (IRB) at research institutions face everyday. An IRB is a committee composed of a diverse group of professionals and laypeople, and is charged with ensuring that human-subjects research in American health-care facilities complies with ethical, legal, and regulatory standards. Since 1974, the U.S. government has mandated that clinical research be reviewed and approved by an IRB that aims to protect human subjects' rights by assessing the risk/benefit ratio of the research and ensuring a valid informed-consent process. Membership of the IRB must include people from diverse backgrounds who have no conflict of interest (financial or otherwise) with the research under review. Rules and procedures by which IRBs at institutions receiving federal funding must operate are described in the U.S. Code of Federal Regulations (Office of Protection from Research Risks, 1994). As IRB members consider the acceptability of research proposals, they must keep in mind that the risks of undertaking research on human subjects must be clear to potential subjects (or to their proxy decision makers) and must be outweighed by potential benefits to the subjects themselves or to other people who have similar conditions (Roberts, Geppert, and Brody 2001).

Development of federal rules and regulations to ensure ethical research methods was inspired in part by the anger and outrage caused by the infamous Tuskegee experiments, in which 400 African-American men in the rural South were followed over several decades (beginning in the 1930s) to observe the progression of their syphilis. Working in a model blindly rooted in scientism, where scientific discovery was valued above all else, the researchers intentionally did not inform the subjects of their disease, provided no treatment (even after penicillin became available in the 1940s), and prevented the subjects from being drafted into the armed forces, where they likely would have been diagnosed and treated appropriately. In response to this tragic abuse, a federal advisory panel was appointed and wrote the Belmont Report, which stated that human-subjects research must adhere to the ethical principles of informed consent, favorable risk/benefit ratios, and fair selection of subjects (National Commission for the Protection of Human Subjects of Biomedical and Behavioral Research, 1981). The U.S. government gave local IRBs the mandate to ensure that these ethical values and federal regulations were implemented meaningfully on the local level where clinical research is conducted.

It is in the day-to-day functioning of the IRB that all the core principles of pragmatism come into play. Clinical investigators are motivated by the wish to acquire new scientific knowledge about psychotropic medications and other interventions that might advance psychiatrists' capacity to diagnose and treat mental disorders. Grant support, patents, and academic advancement often depend on successful conduct of research with human subjects. While the vast majority of medical and psychiatric researchers can balance their personal desire to conduct research with the needs and interests of persons who participate in it, academic zeal may at times cloud their thinking about its possible drawbacks or dangers. More objective individuals, who appreciate the promise and the pitfalls of clinical research, are needed to evaluate its ethical status. Here is where IRBs assume a critical role in addressing ethically sensitive questions about clinical research. Is use of a placebo control justifiable in a study of a new antidepressant medication? Should healthy young children be allowed to serve as the comparison subjects in studies that use powerful magnetic resonance imaging of the brain to study other young children with severe behavioral disturbances? Can subjects be exposed intravenously to drugs of abuse or very high doses of prescribed medications to assess their behavioral and physiological responses? Is it necessary or desirable to inform the potential subjects in an antidepressant medication trial that alternative treatments (such as psychotherapy) are available outside the study and may have a more favorable risk/benefit profile?

As IRB members deliberate the acceptability of clinical research, they must keep in mind that the risks of undertaking research on human subjects must be clear to the potential subjects (or to their proxy decision makers) and must be outweighed by potential benefits to subjects or to others with similar conditions (Pincus, Lieberman, and Ferris 1999). The

IRB fails in its mission if it simply rejects research proposals that carry any risk whatsoever. Human-subjects research always carries some degree of risk, and an overly rigid or uncompromising stance on the part of the IRB could threaten to shut down research projects that in the future might benefit large numbers of people suffering with mental disorders. Such a restriction on psychiatric research would be inconsistent with the mission of academic institutions. Instead, the IRB should work with clinical investigators to ensure development of well-designed studies that can answer pressing clinical questions while guaranteeing protections of informed consent and other ethical imperatives. Interaction between researchers and IRB members ought to be collaborative, non-adversarial, and pragmatically focused.

When all is said and done, psychiatric researchers and IRB members share the same fundamental values: to advance scientific knowledge and to improve treatment options, while protecting people from undue coercion to participate in research and from undue harms that may result from such participation. Clinical pragmatism provides conceptual tools that can help IRB members examine research proposals and consider how best to integrate these scientific, practical, and ethical concerns in order to achieve good outcomes. Pluralism reminds IRB members that there are multiple approaches to understanding and treating mental disorders. It may prompt them to urge psychopharmacology researchers to include study of psychotherapy interventions in their clinical trials—or at least to mention in the consent process that psychotherapy is an alternative or adjunctive treatment. The principle of participatory care highlights the iterative process of informed consent and the need for rigorous, longitudinal assessment of a person's capacity to consent to be part of a study. The IRB may determine that a subject's signing a consent form at the beginning of the study may not be adequate to ensure genuine consent at a later point in the study. Finally, the provisional approach, by taking account of the gradual evolution of science, may lead the IRB to avoid taking an adversarial stance toward investigators but instead work collaboratively with them to design safe and humane research studies that might enhance knowledge in the future. The provisional perspective on psychiatric care may lead the IRB members to encourage researchers to define more clearly (in study protocols and informed-consent documents) how their studies address unanswered questions and might provoke new questions for future investigation.

Scientific research on the human brain and behavior, clinical applications of the findings, and educational programs for young clinicians all are important dimensions of the future of psychiatry. Will psychiatric researchers identify genetic tests that could quantify the risk of developing a mental illness and the likelihood that a specific medication will be effective for that illness? Will brain scans pinpoint the relevant physiological dysfunction underlying a person's manic state or delusional belief, and thereby suggest the necessity of a targeted treatment intervention? Will new medications yet to be discovered be safer and more effective than the helpful but imperfect ones available today? The pragmatic psychiatrist hopes that the answer to these and similar questions is a resounding "yes" and will participate in whatever ways possible to advance the science of psychiatry. But the pragmatic psychiatrist can glimpse the future by careful reflection on the past. No advance in psychiatric neuroscience has ever made people any less complicated than they are or has eliminated the need for understanding them from multiple points of view. As modern neuroscience shows how complex and dynamic the human brain really is, the brain begins to look very much like the human mind, and a lot like human society in general: complicated, perplexing, unpredictable, and elusive. The future of psychiatry lies in fleshing out this complexity while remaining mindful of the fact that the task is daunting and never-ending. And it lies in struggling to find useful new ways to put any available knowledge to work in order to relieve mental and emotional suffering.

Approaches that tend toward the extreme ends of the science/humanism divide fail to meet the everyday needs of the twenty-first-century psychiatrist. Pure humanism in psychiatry runs the risk of shortchanging patients by ignoring scientific knowledge of brain and behavior that may help to relieve emotional suffering. Meanwhile, scientism in psychiatry neglects the existential experience of mental suffering, the multifactorial causation of mental illness, the provisional state of empirical knowledge, and the ethical values that demand that psychiatrists regard patients as fellow human beings and partners in clinical care rather than as scientific specimens. The late Stephen J. Gould (2003, 112) regarded "the concept of oppositional dichotomy between science and the humanities as a foolish negation of our mental capacities and complexities" in the context of the natural sciences in general and evolutionary biology in particular. Likewise, the principal challenge psychiatrists face is to overcome an outdated split between science and humanism that has opened the way for extreme and imprudent theories such as scientism and postmodernism, and to achieve a truly dialectical interplay between science and humanism that is driven by pragmatic reasoning.

The pragmatic psychiatrist must be sensitive to the challenges of the science/humanism divide and strive to heal the conceptual wounds in the field by remaining attuned to the fact that the science of people is (and is likely to remain) a practical, pluralistic, participatory, and provisional science. But pragmatism as an idea and a method of psychiatric reasoning should not be fetishized or set in stone. In fact, turning pragmatism into the one and only model for psychiatric reasoning would be contrary to the open-minded and open-ended values that pragmatism itself espouses. The paradox of philosophical pragmatism is that it calls itself into question continuously. If the pragmatic approach is not working well in everyday life, then it can be discarded in favor of another approach; but that very discarding would be entirely consistent with (and, in fact, demanded by) the pragmatic approach itself. Philosophers and psychiatrists should retain a sense of irony and playfulness about this entire set of ideas. The practicing psychiatrist should adopt clinical pragmatism only insofar as it works to enhance day-to-day patient care. If clinical pragmatism does not work well in a particular case, the psychiatrist should adopt it by rejecting it in favor of a more appealing model and approach to treatment.

A cartoon in *The New Yorker* (June 30, 2003) with the caption "Richard the Pragmatist" depicted a crowned and robed King Richard proclaiming, "My kingdom for a newer, stabler, more centrally located kingdom!" As a theory that is zealous about its moderation, pragmatism lends itself to this kind of spoofing. It is a middle-of-the-road notion that does not grab headlines and is not championed by demagogues. Understanding the extreme nature of its moderation, Menand (2001, 375) wrote that "pragmatism explains everything about ideas except why a person would be willing to die for one." Extreme claims about the promise of science—or its inefficacy—are certainly more likely to generate excitement and brouhaha. Since Foucault, the postmodern rejection of the validity of scientific reasoning (particularly as applied to human experience and behavior) has been very popular in academic and lay literature. At the opposite end of the intellectual spectrum, exuberant faith in the promise of neuroscience for understanding human behavior has continued unabated for many years. How might we ensure that future debates on these subjects are thoughtful and well reasoned but also capture the imaginations of philosophers, psychiatrists, and others who care about understanding the mind and treating people humanely when they are overcome by anxiety, depression, psychosis, and other forms of mental suffering? Can thinkers like "Richard the Pragmatist" be taken seriously and can they generate excitement and passion for their highly practical form of reasoning?

Pragmatic reasoning may not have a great deal of initial sex appeal in the tumultuous marketplace of ideas about human experience and behavior in our times. But while more alluring theories that tend toward extreme ends of the science/humanism spectrum may hold initial appeal, they lose their luster when we examine them carefully and apply them to our everyday needs. Philosopher Charles Taylor (1989, 404) has defined scientism as "the belief that the methods and procedures of natural science suffice to establish all the truths we need to believe"—but he went on to admonish that "nothing assures us that all the issues on which we have to formulate some creed are arbitratable in this fashion. Scientism itself requires a leap of faith." This leap of faith is one that some philosophers and psychiatrists have been all too willing to take, especially when confronted by individuals whose brain dysfunction appears to be the primary cause of their mental illness. Psychiatrists should be reluctant to take the leap of faith into scientism, even when they are diagnosing and treating people with well-defined neuropsychiatric disorders. A more prudent approach at this point in time is to respect the pluralistic and provisional nature of psychiatric explanation and treatment. Clinical cases that I presented throughout the book, from Adam in chapter 3 to Tim in chapter 6, highlight the importance of this point in the real world of everyday psychiatric care.

Still, reaffirming that humanistic approaches in psychiatry continue to have a hold on us in the twenty-first century cannot completely dispel a suspicion that advances in clinical neuroscience, so unimaginable just a few decades ago, might themselves engender further discoveries in future years that will render psychological explanations increasingly obsolete. Even the psychiatrist Robert Coles, whose prolific work teaches us so much about how individual, social, historical, and moral forces shape the human mind (and who never so much as approaches the positions espoused by Wilson and Churchland), cannot help wondering about and being bothered by the idea of reductive materialism in his book *The Secular Mind*. While he recognizes our inability to foresee the details and implications of a "completed neuroscience," Coles (1999, 188) does take seriously the consideration that "the logic of materialism, and our proven capabilities as they inform our restlessly exploring nature, lead us in that direction, foretell our eventual arrival." Yet although he expresses fascination with the conceivability of reductive materialism, Coles speculates in the final pages of his book that a poorly defined notion of selfhood might, in the end, secure a lasting role for a humanistic psychology. We are left not knowing whether to view materialism as a scientistic delusion or a visionary truth-in-the-making.

Object relations theorists, such as Melanie Klein, taught us that young infants split the objects of their experience into purely good and bad objects: the "good breast" nurtures them while the "bad breast" leaves them feeling hungry and uncomfortable. The American pragmatists recognized this troubling tendency as well. "The commonest vice of the human mind," James wrote in *A Pluralistic Universe*, "is its disposition to see everything as yes or no, as black or white, its incapacity for discrimination of intermediate shades" (p. 77–78). Analogously, some philosophers and psychiatrists have tended to regard scientific psychiatry and humanistic psychiatry as either wholly good or wholly bad. There is no doubt that there has been some benefit from the split between science and humanism in psychiatry over the last several decades—for example, the two areas of pursuit would probably never have advanced as far as they did if they had not remained separate. But just as infants take a critical developmental step forward when they recognize that the good and the bad breast are really one and the same object, philosophers and psychiatrists could help their fields mature by recognizing that both scientific and humanistic concepts furnish critical perspectives on the human experience. The traditional dichotomy between science and humanism may be just as untenable (though just as developmentally necessary) as the split that infants experience between a good and a bad breast.

Psychiatrists face the task of working through and hopefully healing the split in our vision of what makes people feel and act as they do, whether in illness or in health. The divide between science and humanism has become burdensome and self-defeating. The major developmental challenge psychiatrists face as we move forward in the new century is to push beyond the current position, where an unworkable split between empirical science and humanistic psychology opens the way for captivating but extreme and imprudent theories like scientism and postmodernism. These theories are intellectually intriguing but are methodologically useless for patients who cannot be understood or treated effectively in the terms of a single psychiatric explanatory model, but whose suffering may be quite understandable and treatable if it is approached in a multidimensional, flexible, collaborative, and open-ended manner. The twenty-first-century psychiatrist needs to aim toward a position where a dialectical interaction between science and humanism, informed and motored by a pragmatic ethic, is not only tolerated but is used in an exciting and constructive way—and where an unabashed effort to hold onto and to integrate a diversity of human phenomena urges psychiatry forward to a new day.

References

Agich, G.J. 2002. Implications of a pragmatic theory of disease for the DSMs. In J.Z. Sadler, ed. *Descriptions and Prescriptions: Values, Mental Disorders, and the DSMs*, 96–113. Baltimore: Johns Hopkins University Press.

American Psychiatric Association. 1952. *Diagnostic and Statistical Manual of Mental Disorders*. (DSM-I.) Washington, DC: American Psychiatric Association.

American Psychiatric Association. 1968. *Diagnostic and Statistical Manual of Mental Disorders*. 2nd ed. (DSM-II.) Washington, DC: American Psychiatric Association.

American Psychiatric Association. 1980. *Diagnostic and Statistical Manual of Mental Disorders*. 3rd ed. (DSM-III.) Washington, DC: American Psychiatric Association.

American Psychiatric Association. 1987. *Diagnostic and Statistical Manual of Mental Disorders*. 3rd ed., rev. (DSM-III-R.) Washington, DC: American Psychiatric Association.

American Psychiatric Association. 1994. *Diagnostic and Statistical Manual of Mental Disorders*. 4th ed. (DSM-IV.) Washington, DC: American Psychiatric Association.

American Psychiatric Association. 2000. *Diagnostic and Statistical Manual of Mental Disorders*. 4th ed., text revision. (DSM-IV-TR.) Washington, DC: American Psychiatric Association.

Arieti, S. 1972. Volition and value: A study based on catatonic schizophrenia. In S. C. Post, ed., *Moral Values and the Superego Concept in Psycho-analysis*, 275–288. New York: International Universities Press.

Arras, J. D. 2003. Rorty's pragmatism and bioethics. *Journal of Medicine and Philosophy* 28:597–613.

Bader, M. J. 1994. The tendency to neglect therapeutic aims in psychoanalysis. *Psychoanalytic Quarterly* 63:246–270.

Baxter, L. R., Schwartz, J. M., Bergman, K. S., et al. 1992. Caudate glucose metabolic rate changes with both drug and behavior therapy for obsessive-compulsive disorder. *Archives of General Psychiatry* 49:681–689.

Bayer, R., and Spitzer, R. L. 1985. Neurosis, psychodynamics, and DSM-III: A history of the controversy. *Archives of General Psychiatry* 42:187–196.

Bellantoni, L. 2003. What good is a pragmatic bioethic? *Journal of Medicine and Philosophy* 28:615–633.

Bernfield, S. 1944. Freud's earliest theories and the school of Helmholtz. *Psychoanalytic Quarterly* 13:341–361.

Bernstein, R. J. 1988. Pragmatism, pluralism, and the healing of wounds. In L. Menand, ed., *Pragmatism: A reader,* 382–401. New York: Vintage Books, 1997.

Bloch, S., Chodoff, P., and Green, S. A., eds. 1999. *Psychiatric Ethics.* 3rd ed. Oxford: Oxford University Press.

Bolton, D. 1997. Encoding of meaning: Deconstructing the meaning/causality distinction. *Philosophy, Psychiatry, & Psychology* 4:255–267.

Bolton, D., and Hill, J. 1996. *Mind, Meaning, and Mental Disorder: The Nature of Causal Explanation in Psychology and Psychiatry.* Oxford: Oxford University Press.

Bracken, P., and Thomas, P. 2001. Postpsychiatry: A new direction for mental health. *British Medical Journal* 322:724–727.

Braslow, J. T. 1995. Effect of therapeutic innovation on perception of disease and the doctor-patient relationship: A history of general paralysis of the insane and malaria fever therapy, 1910–1950. *American Journal of Psychiatry* 152:660–665.

Brendel, D. H. 2000. Philosophy of mind in the clinic: The relation between causal and meaningful explanation in psychiatry. *Harvard Review of Psychiatry* 8:184–191.

Brendel, D. H. 2001. Multifactorial causation of mental disorders: A proposal to improve the DSM. *Harvard Review of Psychiatry* 9:42–45.

Brendel, D. H. 2002. The ethics of diagnostic and therapeutic paradigm choice in psychiatry. *Harvard Review of Psychiatry* 10:47–50.

Brendel, D. H. 2003a. Complications to consent. *Journal of Clinical Ethics* 14:90–94.

Brendel, D. H. 2003b. A pragmatic consideration of the relation between depression and melancholia. *Philosophy, Psychiatry, & Psychology* 10:53–55.

Brendel, D. H. 2003c. Reductionism, eclecticism, and pragmatism in psychiatry: The dialectic of clinical explanation. *Journal of Medicine and Philosophy* 28:563–580.

Brendel, D. H. 2004. Healing psychiatry: A pragmatic approach to bridging the science/humanism divide. *Harvard Review of Psychiatry* 12:150–157.

Brendel, D. H., Bodkin, J. A., Hauptman, B., and Ornstein, A. 2002. "I see dead people": Overcoming psychic numbness. *Harvard Review of Psychiatry* 10:166–178.

Brendel, D. H., Florman, J., Roberts, S., and Solet, J. M. 2001. "In sleep I almost never grope": Blindness, neuropsychiatric deficits, and a chaotic upbringing. *Harvard Review of Psychiatry* 9:178–188.

Breuer, J. 1893–1895. Studies on hysteria case 1: Fräulein Anna O. In S. Freud, *The Standard Edition of the Complete Psychological Works of Sigmund Freud,* trans. J Strachey, vol. 2, pp. 21–47. London: Hogarth Press, 1955.

Brock, D. W. 1991. The ideal of shared decision making between physicians and patients. *Kennedy Institute of Ethics Journal* 1:28–47.

Bruyer, R. 1991. Covert face recognition in prosopagnosia: A review. *Brain and Cognition* 15:223–235.

Bunge, M. 1977. Emergence and the mind. *Neuroscience* 2:501–509.

Busch, F. N., Cooper, A. M., Klerman, G. L., Penzer, R. J., Shapiro, T., and Shear, M. K. 1991. Neurophysiological, cognitive-behavioral, and psychoanalytic approaches to panic disorder: Toward an integration. *Psychoanalytic Inquiry* 11:316–332.

Carey, B. 2004. For psychotherapy's claims, skeptics demand proof. *New York Times,* August 10, sec. F, p. 1, col. 1.

Carroll, B. T., Anfinson, T. J., Kennedy, J. C., Yendrek, R., Boutros, M., and Bilon, A. 1994. Catatonic disorder due to general medical conditions. *Journal of Neuropsychiatry and Clinical Neurosciences* 6:122–133.

Carter, J. 2003. Looking into a distorted mirror. *Journal of Clinical Ethics* 14:95–100.

Carter, M. A. 2000. A synthetic approach to bioethical inquiry. *Theoretical Medicine* 21:217–234.

Chabolla, D. R., Krahn, L. E., So, E. L., and Rummans, T. A. 1996. Psychogenic nonepileptic seizures. *Mayo Clinic Proceedings* 71:493–500.

Chalmers, D. J. 1996. *The conscious mind: In search of a fundamental theory.* New York: Oxford University Press.

Churchland, P. M. 1981. Eliminative materialism and propositional attitudes. *Journal of Philosophy* 78:67–90.

Churchland, P. M. 1988. *Matter and Consciousness: A Contemporary Introduction to the Philosophy of Mind.* Cambridge, MA: MIT Press.

Churchland, P. M. 1995. *The Engine of Reason, the Seat of the Soul: A Philosophical Journey into the Brain.* Cambridge, MA: MIT Press.

Coles, R. 1999. *The Secular Mind.* Princeton, NJ: Princeton University Press.

Cooke, E. F. 2003. On the possibility of a pragmatic discourse bioethics: Putnam, Habermas, and the normative logic of bioethical inquiry. *Journal of Medicine and Philosophy* 28:635–653.

Corbí, J. E., and Prades, J. L. 2000. *Minds, Causes, and Mechanisms: A Case against Physicalism.* Oxford: Blackwell.

Damasio, A. R. 1994. *Descartes' Error: Emotion, Reason, and the Human Brain.* New York: Putnam.

Darwin, C. 1859. *On the Origin of Species by Means of Natural Selection, or the Preservation of Favoured Races in the Struggle for Life.* London: John Murray.

Daston, L. 1982. The theory of will versus the science of mind. In W. R. Woodward and M. G. Ash, eds., *The Problematic Science: Psychology in Nineteenth-Century Thought,* 88–115. New York: Praeger.

Davidson, D. 1980. Mental events. In D. Davidson, *Essays on Actions and Events,* 207–227. Oxford: Clarendon Press.

Dewey, J. 1917. The need for a recovery of philosophy. In J. A. Boydston, ed., *The Middle Works,* vol. 10. Carbondale, IL: Southern Illinois University Press, 1978.

Dewey, J. 1925. Experience and nature. In J. A. Boydston, ed., *The Later Works,* vol. 1. Carbondale, IL: Southern Illinois University Press, 1985.

Dewey, J. 1929. The quest for certainty: A study of the relation of knowledge and action. In J. A. Boydston, ed., *The Later Works,* vol. 4. Carbondale, IL: Southern Illinois University Press, 1985.

Dewhurst, D., and Watson, I. P. B. 1996. Unity and diversity in psychiatry: Some philosophical issues. *Australian and New Zealand Journal of Psychiatry* 30:382–388.

Dickersin, K., and Rennie, D. 2003. Registering clinical trials. *Journal of the American Medical Association* 290:516–523.

Dickstein, M., ed. 1998. *The Revival of Pragmatism: New Essays on Social Thought, Law, and Culture.* Durham, NC: Duke University Press.

Diggins, J. P. 1994. *The Promise of Pragmatism: Modernism and the Crisis of Knowledge and Authority.* Chicago: University of Chicago Press.

Doidge, N. 1997. Empirical evidence for the efficacy of psychoanalytic psychotherapies and psychoanalysis: An overview. *Psychoanalytic Inquiry* (suppl.): 102–150.

Dupré, J. 1993. *The Disorder of Things: Metaphysical Foundations of the Disunity of Science.* Cambridge, MA: Harvard University Press.

Eccles, J. 1973. *The Understanding of the Brain.* New York: McGraw-Hill.

Eisenberg, L. 1986. Mindlessness and brainlessness in psychiatry. *British Journal of Psychiatry* 148:497–508.

Eisenberg, L. 1995. The social construction of the human brain. *American Journal of Psychiatry* 152:1563–1575.

Engel, G. 1977. The need for a new medical model: A challenge for biomedicine. *Science* 196:129–136.

Engel, G. 1980. The clinical application of the biopsychosocial model. *American Journal of Psychiatry* 137:535–544.

Epstein, R. M. 1999. Mindful practice. *Journal of the American Medical Association* 282:833–839.

Expert Consensus Panels for PTSD. 1999. *Journal of Clinical Psychiatry* 60 (suppl. 16):3–76.

Fins, J. J., Bacchetta, M. D., and Miller, F. G. 1997. Clinical pragmatism: A method of moral problem solving. *Kennedy Institute of Ethics Journal* 7:129–143.

Fins, J. J., Miller, F. G., and Bacchetta, M. D. 1998. Clinical pragmatism: Bridging theory and practice. *Kennedy Institute of Ethics Journal* 8:37–42.

Fogel, B. S. 1990. Major depression versus organic mood disorder: A questionable distinction. *Journal of Clinical Psychiatry* 51:53–56.

Follette, W. C., and Houts, A. C. 1996. Models of scientific progress and the role of theory in taxonomy development: A case study of the DSM. *Journal of Consulting and Clinical Psychology* 64:1120–1132.

Foucault, M. 1965. *Madness and Civilization: A History of Insanity in the Age of Reason.* New York: Pantheon.

Frattaroli, E. 2001. *Healing the Soul in the Age of the Brain: Why Medication Isn't Enough.* New York: Penguin Books.

Freud, S. 1884. A new histological method for the study of nerve tracts in the brain and spinal cord. *Brain* 7:86–89.

Freud, S. 1886. Observation of a severe case of hemi-anaesthesia in a hysterical male. In S. Freud, *The Standard Edition of the Complete Psychological Works of Sigmund Freud,* trans. J. Strachey, vol. 1, pp. 25–31. London: Hogarth Press, 1955.

Freud, S. 1887. Two short reviews. In S. Freud, *The Standard Edition of the Complete Psychological Works of Sigmund Freud,* trans. J. Strachey, vol. 1, pp. 35–36. London: Hogarth Press, 1955.

Freud, S. 1891. *On Aphasia,* trans. E. Stengel. New York: International Universities Press, 1953.

Freud, S. 1893. Some points for a comparative study of organic and hysterical motor paralyses. In S. Freud, *The Standard Edition of the Complete Psychological Works of Sigmund Freud,* trans. J. Strachey, vol. 1, pp. 160–172. London: Hogarth Press, 1955.

Freud, S. 1893–1895. Studies on hysteria case 5: Fräulein Elisabeth von R. In S. Freud, *The Standard Edition of the Complete Psychological Works of Sigmund Freud,* trans. J. Strachey, vol. 2, pp. 135–181. London: Hogarth Press, 1955.

Freud, S. 1894. The neuro-psychoses of defense. In S. Freud, *The Standard Edition of the Complete Psychological Works of Sigmund Freud,* trans. J. Strachey, vol. 3, pp. 45–61. London: Hogarth Press, 1955.

Freud, S. 1905a. Fragment of an analysis of a case of hysteria. In S. Freud, *The Standard Edition of the Complete Psychological Works of Sigmund Freud,* trans. J. Strachey, vol. 7, pp. 7–122. London: Hogarth Press, 1955.

Freud, S. 1905b. Psychical (or mental) treatment. In S. Freud, *The Standard Edition of the Complete Psychological Works of Sigmund Freud,* trans. J. Strachey, vol. 7, pp. 283–302. London: Hogarth Press, 1955.

Freud, S. 1909. Notes upon a case of obsessional neurosis. In S. Freud, *The Standard Edition of the Complete Psychological Works of Sigmund Freud,* trans. J. Strachey, vol. 10, pp. 155–318. London: Hogarth Press, 1955.

Freud, S. 1914a. On the history of the psycho-analytic movement. In S. Freud, *The Standard Edition of the Complete Psychological Works of Sigmund Freud,* trans. J. Strachey, vol. 14, pp. 1–66. London: Hogarth Press, 1955.

Freud, S. 1914b. Remembering, repeating, and working-through. In S. Freud, *The Standard Edition of the Complete Psychological Works of Sigmund Freud,* trans. J. Strachey, vol. 12, pp. 145–156. London: Hogarth Press, 1955.

Freud, S. 1915a. Observations on transference-love. In S. Freud, *The Standard Edition of the Complete Psychological Works of Sigmund Freud,* trans. J. Strachey, vol. 12, pp. 157–173. London: Hogarth Press, 1955.

Freud, S. 1915b. The unconscious. In S. Freud, *The Standard Edition of the Complete Psychological Works of Sigmund Freud,* trans. J. Strachey, vol. 14, pp. 166–204. London: Hogarth Press, 1955.

Freud, S. 1920. Beyond the pleasure principle. In S. Freud, *The Standard Edition of the Complete Psychological Works of Sigmund Freud,* trans. J. Strachey, vol. 18, pp. 7–64. London: Hogarth Press, 1955.

Freud, S. 1925. An autobiographical study. In S. Freud, *The Standard Edition of the Complete Psychological Works of Sigmund Freud,* trans. J. Strachey, vol. 20, pp. 7–74. London: Hogarth Press, 1955.

Freud, S. 1927. The future of an illusion. In S. Freud, *The Standard Edition of the Complete Psychological Works of Sigmund Freud,* trans. J. Strachey, vol. 21, pp. 5–56. London: Hogarth Press, 1955.

Freud, S. 1933. The question of a *Weltanschauung.* In S. Freud, *The Standard Edition of the Complete Psychological Works of Sigmund Freud,* trans. J. Strachey, vol. 22, pp. 158–182. London: Hogarth Press, 1955.

Freud, S. 1937. Analysis terminable and interminable. In S. Freud, *The Standard Edition of the Complete Psychological Works of Sigmund Freud,* trans. J. Strachey, vol. 23, pp. 209–253. London: Hogarth Press, 1955.

Fulford, K. W. M. 1999. Analytic philosophy, brain science, and the concept of disorder. In S. Bloch, S. P. Chodoff, and S. A. Green, eds., *Psychiatric Ethics,* 3rd ed., 161–191. Oxford: Oxford University Press.

Fulford, K. W. M., and Hope, T. 1994. Psychiatric ethics: A bioethical ugly duckling? In R. Gillon, ed., *Principles of Health Care Ethics,* 681–695. New York: Wiley.

Gabbard, G. O. 1992. Psychodynamic psychiatry in the "decade of the brain." *American Journal of Psychiatry* 149:991–998.

Gabbard, G. O., and Kay, J. 2001. The fate of integrated treatment: Whatever happened to the biopsychosocial psychiatrist? *American Journal of Psychiatry* 158:1956–1963.

Gabbard, G. O., Lazar, S. G., Hornberger, J., and Speigel, D. 1997. The economic impact of psychotherapy: A review. *American Journal of Psychiatry* 154:147–155.

Gawande, A. 2002. *Complications: A surgeon's notes on an imperfect science.* New York: Holt.

Gay, P. 1988. *Freud: A Life for Our Time.* New York: Doubleday.

Geschwind, N. 1975. The borderland of neurology and psychiatry: some common misconceptions. In D. F. Benson and D. Blumer, eds., *Psychiatric Aspects of Neurologic Disease,* vol. 1, pp. 1–8. New York: Grune & Stratton.

Ghaemi, S. N. 2003. *The Concepts of Psychiatry: A Pluralistic Approach to the Mind and Mental Illness.* Baltimore: Johns Hopkins University Press.

Goldberg, A. 2002. American pragmatism and American psychoanalysis. *Psychoanalytic Quarterly* 71:235–254.

Gorman, J. M., Liebowitz, M.R., Fyer, A. J., and Stein, J. 1989. A neuroanatomical hypothesis for panic disorder. *American Journal of Psychiatry* 146:148–161.

Gould, S. J. 2003. *The Hedgehog, the Fox, and the Magister's Pox: Mending the Gap between Science and the Humanities.* New York: Harmony Books.

Green, S. A., and Bloch, S. 2001. Working in a flawed mental health care system: An ethical challenge. *American Journal of Psychiatry* 158:1378–1383.

Guze, S. B. 1989. Biological psychiatry: Is there any other kind? *Psychological Medicine* 19:315–323.

Halpern, J. 2003. Beyond wishful thinking: Facing the harm that psychotherapists can do by writing about their patients. *Journal of Clinical Ethics* 14:118–136.

Hare, E. H. 1959. The origin and spread of dementia paralytica. *Journal of Mental Science* 105:594–626.

Hart, C. W. 2002. Helen Flanders Dunbar, John Dewey, and clinical pragmatism: Reflections on method in psychosomatic medicine and bioethics. *Journal of Pastoral Care & Counseling* 56:265–269.

Havens, L. L. 1973. *Approaches to the Mind: Movement of the Psychiatric Schools from Sects toward Science.* Boston: Little, Brown.

Hegel, G. W. F. 1977. *The Phenomenology of Spirit,* trans. A. V. Miller. Oxford: Oxford University Press.

Hester, D. M. 2003. Is pragmatism well-suited to bioethics? *Journal of Medicine and Philosophy* 28:545–561.

Hoffman, I. Z. 1994. Dialectical thinking and therapeutic action in the psychoanalytic process. *Psychoanalytic Quarterly* 63:187–218.

Holt, R. R. 2002. Postmodernism: Its origin and its threat to psychoanalysis. *International Forum of Psychoanalysis* 11:264–274.

Horgan, T. 1993. Nonreductive materialism and the explanatory autonomy of psychology. In S. J. Warner and R. Warner, eds., *Naturalism: A Critical Appraisal,* 295–320. Notre Dame, IN: University of Notre Dame Press.

Howe, E. G. 2003. Lessons from "Jay Carter." *Journal of Clinical Ethics* 14:109–117.

Hudson, J. I., and Pope, H. G., Jr. 1990. Affective spectrum disorder: Does antidepressant response identify a family of disorders with a common pathophysiology? *American Journal of Psychiatry* 147:552–564.

Hundert, E. M. 1989. *Philosophy, Psychiatry, and Neuroscience: Three Approaches to the Mind.* Oxford: Oxford University Press.

Hundert, E. M. 1992. The brain's capacity to form delusions as an evolutionary strategy for survival. In M. Spitzer, F. A. Uehlein, M. A. Schwartz, and C. Mundt, eds., *Phenomenology, Language, & Schizophrenia,* 346–354. New York: Springer.

James, W. 1909. *A Pluralistic Universe.* Lincoln, NE: University of Nebraska Press, 1996.

James, W. 1904. Humanism and truth. In W. James, *Pragmatism and the Meaning of Truth,* 203–226. Cambridge, MA: Harvard University Press, 1975.

James, W. 1906. The one and the many. In W. James, *Pragmatism and the Meaning of Truth,* 63–79. Cambridge, MA: Harvard University Press, 1975.

James, W. 1890. *The Principles of Psychology.* New York: Holt.

James, W. 1901–1902. *The Varieties of Religious Experience.* New York: Touchstone, 1997.

James, W. 1907. What pragmatism means. In W. James, *Essays in Pragmatism,* 141–158. New York: Hafner Press, 1948.

Jansen, L. A. 1998. Assessing clinical pragmatism. *Kennedy Institute of Ethics Journal* 8:23–36.

Jaspers, K. 1913. *General Psychopathology.* Baltimore: Johns Hopkins University Press, 1997.

Joffe, S. 2003. Public dialogue and the boundaries of moral community. *Journal of Clinical Ethics* 14:101–108.

Kandel, E. R. 1979. Psychotherapy and the single synapse: The impact of psychiatric thought on neurobiologic research. *New England Journal of Medicine* 301:1028–1037.

Kandel, E. R. 1998. A new intellectual framework for psychiatry. *American Journal of Psychiatry* 155:457–469.

Karlsson, H., and Kamppinen, M. 1995. Biological psychiatry and reductionism: Empirical findings and philosophy. *British Journal of Psychiatry* 167:434–438.

Keller, M. B., McCullough, J. P., Klein, D. N., Arnow, B., Dunner, D. L., Gelenberg, A. J., Markowitz, J. C., Nemeroff, C. B., Russell, J. M., Thase, M. E., Trivedi, M. H., and Zajecka, J. 2000. A comparison of nefazodone, the cognitive-behavioral analysis system of psychotherapy, and their combination for the treatment of chronic depression. *New England Journal of Medicine* 342:1462–1470.

Kendler, K. S., Karkowski, L. M., and Prescott, C. A. 1999. Causal relationship between stressful life events and the onset of major depression. *American Journal of Psychiatry* 156:837–841.

Kim, J. 1996. *Philosophy of Mind.* Boulder, CO: Westview Press.

Klerman, G. L. 1990. The psychiatric patient's right to effective treatment: Implications of *Osheroff v. Chestnut Lodge*. *American Journal of Psychiatry* 147:409–418.

Klerman, G. L., Endicott, J., Spitzer, R., and Hirschfeld, R. M. A. 1979. Neurotic depressions: A systematic analysis of multiple criteria and meanings. *American Journal of Psychiatry* 136:57–61.

Klerman, G. L., Vaillant, G. E., Spitzer, R. L., and Michels, R. 1984. A debate on DSM-III. *American Journal of Psychiatry* 141:539–553.

Kopin, I. J. 1993. Parkinson's disease: Past, present, and future. *Neuropsychopharmacology* 9:1–12.

Lazare, A. 1973. Hidden conceptual models in clinical psychiatry. *New England Journal of Medicine* 288:345–351.

Lear, J. 2000. *Happiness, Death, and the Remainder of Life*. Cambridge, MA: Harvard University Press.

Lee, B. X., and Wexler, B. E. 1999. Physics and the quandaries of contemporary psychiatry: Review and research. *Psychiatry* 62:222–234.

Leff, J., and Vaughn, C. 1985. *Expressed Emotion in Families: Its Significance for Mental Illness*. New York: Guilford.

Leis, A. A., Ross, M. A., and Summers, A. K. 1992. Psychogenic seizures: Ictal characteristics and diagnostic pitfalls. *Neurology* 42:95–99.

Lewis, B. L. 2000. Psychiatry and postmodern theory. *Journal of Medical Humanities* 21:71–84.

Lewontin, R. 2001. After the genome, what then? *New York Review of Books* 48(12):36–37.

Luhrmann, T. M. 2000. *Of Two Minds: The Growing Disorder in American Psychiatry*. New York: Knopf.

Lyoo, I. K., Seol, H. Y., Byun, H. S., and Renshaw, P. F. 1996. Unsuspected multiple sclerosis in patients with psychiatric disorders: A magnetic resonance imaging study. *Journal of Neuropsychiatry and Clinical Neurosciences* 8:54–59.

Macdonald, G. 1995. Introduction: Psychoanalytic explanation. In C. Macdonald and G. Macdonald, eds., *Philosophy of Psychology: Debates on Psychological Explanation*, 394–408. Oxford: Blackwell.

Martin, J. B. 2002. The integration of neurology, psychiatry, and neuroscience in the 21st century. *American Journal of Psychiatry* 159:695–704.

Martin, P. A. 1999. Bioethics and the whole: Pluralism, consensus, and the transmutation of bioethical methods into gold. *Journal of Law, Medicine, & Ethics* 27:316–327.

McCauley, R. N. 1996. Explanatory pluralism and the co-evolution of theories in science. In R. N. McCauley, ed., *The Churchlands and Their Critics*, 17–47. Cambridge, MA: Blackwell.

McGee, G., ed. 2003. *Pragmatic Bioethics*. 2nd ed. Cambridge, MA: MIT Press.

McGinn, C. 1994. Can we solve the mind-body problem? In R. Warner and T. Szubka, eds., *The Mind-Body Problem: A Guide to the Current Debate*, 99–120. Cambridge, MA: Blackwell.

McHugh, P. R., and Slavney, P. R. 1998. *The Perspectives of Psychiatry*. 2nd ed. Baltimore: Johns Hopkins University Press.

McLaren, N. 1998. A critical review of the biopsychosocial model. *Australian and New Zealand Journal of Psychiatry* 32:86–92.

Menand, L. 2001. *The Metaphysical Club: A Story of Ideas in America*. New York: Farrar, Straus, and Giroux.

Miller, F. G., Fins, J. J., and Bacchetta, M. D. 1996. Clinical pragmatism: John Dewey and clinical ethics. *Journal of Contemporary Health Law and Policy* 13:27–51.

Miller, L. 1991. *Freud's Brain: Neuropsychodynamic Foundations of Psychoanalysis*. New York: Guilford.

Milrod, B., Busch, F. N., Hollander, E., Aronson, A., and Siever, L. 1996. A 23-year-old woman with panic disorder treated with psychodynamic psychotherapy. *American Journal of Psychiatry* 153:698–703.

Mitchell, C., and Truog, R. 2003. Seeking blinded consent. *Journal of Clinical Ethics* 14:88–89.

Nagel, T. 1974. What is it like to be a bat? *Philosophical Review* 83:435–450.

National Commission for the Protection of Human Subjects of Biomedical and Behavioral Research. 1981. *The Belmont Report: Ethical Principles and Guidelines for the Protection of Human Subjects of Research*. Washington, DC: U.S. Government Printing Office.

Nemiah, J. 1981. The idea of a psychiatric education. *Journal of Psychiatric Education* 5:183–194.

Nesse, R. M. 2000. Is depression an adaptation? *Archives of General Psychiatry* 57:14–20.

Office of Protection from Research Risks. 1994. *OPRR Reports: Protection of Human Subjects*. Title 45 Code of Federal Regulations, Part 46. Washington, DC: U.S. Government Printing Office.

Olafson, F. A. 2001. *Naturalism and the Human Condition: Against Scientism*. New York: Routledge.

Parascandola, M., Hawkins, J., and Danis, M. 2002. Patient autonomy and the challenge of clinical uncertainty. *Kennedy Institute of Ethics Journal* 12:245–264.

Paykel, E. S. 1978. Contribution of life events to causation of psychiatric illness. *Psychological Medicine* 8:245–253.

Peirce, C. S. 1890. A guess at the riddle. In L. Menand, ed., *Pragmatism: A Reader*, 49–51. New York: Vintage Books, 1997.

Peirce, C. S. 1904. A definition of pragmatism. In L. Menand, ed., *Pragmatism: A Reader*, 56–58. New York: Vintage Books, 1997.

Perry, S., Cooper, A. M., and Michels, R. 1987. The psychodynamic formulation: Its purpose, structure, and clinical application. *American Journal of Psychiatry* 144:543–550.

Pincus, H. A., Lieberman, J. A., and Ferris, S., eds. 1999. *Ethics in Psychiatric Research: A Resource Manual for Human Subjects Protection.* Washington, DC: American Psychiatric Association.

Price, B. H., Adams, R. D., and Coyle, J. T. 2000. Neurology and psychiatry: Closing the great divide. *Neurology* 54:8–14.

Putnam, H. 1999. *The Threefold Cord: Mind, Body, and World.* New York: Columbia University Press.

Quetel, C. 1990. *History of Syphilis.* Baltimore: Johns Hopkins University Press.

Radden, J. 2003. Is this dame melancholy? Equating today's depression and past melancholia. *Philosophy, Psychiatry, & Psychology* 10:37–52.

Rescher, N. 2000. *Realistic Pragmatism: An Introduction to Pragmatic Philosophy.* Albany, NY: State University of New York Press.

Roberts, G. 1991. Delusional belief systems and meaning in life: A preferred reality? *British Journal of Psychiatry* 159(suppl. 14):19–28.

Roberts, L. W., Geppert, C. M. A., and Brody, J. L. 2001. A framework for considering the ethical aspects of psychiatric research protocols. *Comprehensive Psychiatry* 42:351–363.

Robertson, M. M., and Yakely, J. 1996. Gilles de la Tourette syndrome and obsessive-compulsive disorder. In B. S. Fogel and R. B. Schiffer, eds., *Neuropsychiatry,* 827–870. Baltimore: Williams & Wilkins.

Rogers, D. 1991. Catatonia: A contemporary approach. *Journal of Neuropsychiatry and Clinical Neurosciences* 3:334–340.

Rorty, R. 1979. *Philosophy and the Mirror of Nature.* Princeton, NJ: Princeton University Press.

Rorty, R. 1982. Pragmatism, relativism, and irrationalism. In R. Rorty, *Consequences of Pragmatism,* 160–175. Minneapolis: University of Minnesota Press.

Rosenthal, S. B., Hausman, C. R., and Anderson, D. R., eds. 1999. *Classical American Pragmatism: Its Contemporary Vitality.* Urbana: University of Illinois Press.

Roth, M., and Kroll, J. 1986. *The Reality of Mental Illness.* Cambridge: Cambridge University Press.

Roy, A. 1989. Pseudoseizures: A psychiatric perspective. *Journal of Neuropsychiatry and Clinical Neurosciences* 1:69–71.

Rudnick, A. 2002. The molecular turn in psychiatry: A philosophical analysis. *Journal of Medicine and Philosophy* 27:287–296.

Sadler, J. Z. 1997. Recognizing values: A descriptive-causal method for medical/scientific discourses. *Journal of Medicine and Philosophy* 22:541–565.

Sadler, J. Z. 2004. *Values and Psychiatric Diagnosis.* New York: Oxford University Press.

Sadler, J. Z., ed. 2002. *Descriptions and Prescriptions: Values, Mental Disorders, and the DSMs.* Baltimore: Johns Hopkins University Press.

Sadler, J. Z., Hulgus, Y. F., and Agich, G. J. 1994. On values in recent American psychiatric classification. *Journal of Medicine and Philosophy* 19:266–277.

Sano, M., Stern, Y., Cote, L., Williams, J. B., and Mayeux, R. 1990. Depression in Parkinson's disease: A biochemical model. *Journal of Neuropsychiatry and Clinical Neurosciences* 2:88–92.

Saygi, S., Deniz, G., Kutsal, O., and Vural, N. 1992. Frontal lobe partial seizures and psychogenic seizures: Comparison of clinical and ictal characteristics. *Neurology* 42:1274–1277.

Schafer, M. 1999. Nomothetic and idiographic methodology in psychiatry—a historical-philosophical analysis. *Medicine, Health Care, and Philosophy* 2:265–274.

Schlenger, W. E., Caddell, J. M., Ebert, L., Jordan, B. K., Rourke, K. M., Wilson, D., Thalji, L., Dennis, J. M., Fairbank, J. A., and Kulka, R. A. 2002. Psychological reactions to terrorist attacks: Findings from the National Study of Americans' Reactions to September 11. *Journal of the American Medical Association* 288:581–588.

Schmidt-Felzmann, H. 2003. Pragmatic principles—methodological pluralism in the principle-based approach to bioethics. *Journal of Medicine and Philosophy* 28:581–596.

Schön, D. A. 1983. *The Reflective Practitioner: How Professionals Think in Action.* New York: Basic Books.

Schwartz, M. A., and Wiggins, O. P. 1985. Science, humanism, and the nature of medical practice: A phenomenological view. *Perspectives in Biology and Medicine* 28:331–366.

Servan-Schreiber, D. 2004. *The Instinct to Heal: Curing Stress, Anxiety, and Depression without Drugs and without Talk Therapy.* New York: St. Martin's Press.

Sider, R. C. 1984. The ethics of therapeutic modality choice. *American Journal of Psychiatry* 141:390–394.

Smith, J. E. 1999. Introduction. In S. B. Rosenthal, C. R Hausman, and D. R. Anderson, eds., *Classical American Pragmatism: Its Contemporary Vitality,* 1–11. Urbana: University of Illinois Press.

Spitzer, R. L., First, M. B., Williams, J. B., Kendler, K., Pincus, H. A., and Tucker, G. 1992. Now is the time to retire the term "organic mental disorders." *American Journal of Psychiatry* 149:240–244.

Stone, A. A. 1990. Law, science, and psychiatric malpractice: A response to Klerman's indictment of psychoanalytic psychiatry. *American Journal of Psychiatry* 147:419–427.

Stone, A. A. 2001. Psychotherapy in the managed care health market. *Journal of Psychiatric Practice* 7:238–243.

Strachey, J. 1893. Editor's note. In J. Strachey, ed. and trans., *The Standard Edition of the Complete Psychological Works of Sigmund Freud*, vol. 1, pp. 157–159. London: Hogarth Press, 1955.

Sullivan, M. D. 1990. Organic or functional? Why psychiatry needs a philosophy of mind. *Psychiatric Annals* 20:271–277.

Swanson, J. W., Tepper, M. C., Backlar, P., and Swartz, M. S. 2000. Psychiatric advance directives: An alternative to coercive treatment? *Psychiatry* 63:160–172.

Taylor, A. E., and Saint-Cyr, J. A. 1990. Depression in Parkinson's disease: Reconciling physiological and psychological perspectives. *Journal of Neuropsychiatry and Clinical Neurosciences* 2:92–98.

Taylor, C. 1985. How is mechanism conceivable? In C. Taylor, *Human Agency and Language*, 45–76. Cambridge: Cambridge University Press.

Taylor, C. 1989. *Sources of the Self*. Cambridge, MA: Harvard University Press.

Tollefsen, C. 2000. What would John Dewey do? The promises and perils of pragmatic bioethics. *Journal of Medicine and Philosophy* 25:77–106.

Tollefsen, C., and Cherry, M. J. 2003. Pragmatism and bioethics: Diagnosis or cure? *Journal of Medicine and Philosophy* 28:533–544.

Trotter, G. 2003. Pragmatic bioethics and the big fat moral community. *Journal of Medicine and Philosophy* 28:655–671.

Vaughan, S. C. 1997. *The Talking Cure: The Science Behind Psychotherapy*. New York: Putnam.

Wallerstein, R. 1994. Foreword. In G. O Gabbard, ed., *Psychodynamic Psychiatry in Clinical Practice: The DSM-IV Edition*, ix–xii. Washington, DC: American Psychiatric Press.

Warner, R., and Szubka, T. 1994. *The Mind-Body Problem: A Guide to the Current Debate*. Cambridge, MA: Blackwell.

Weinberg, S. 2001. Can science explain everything? Anything? *New York Review of Books* 48(9):47–50.

Westen, D. 1998. The scientific legacy of Sigmund Freud: Toward a psychodynamically informed psychological science. *Psychological Bulletin* 124:333–371.

Westen, D. 2002. Implications of developments in cognitive neuroscience for psychoanalytic psychotherapy. *Harvard Review of Psychiatry* 10:369–373.

Westen, D., Novotny, C. M., and Thompson-Brenner, H. 2004. The empirical status of empirically supported psychotherapies: Assumptions, findings, and reporting in controlled clinical trials. *Psychological Bulletin* 130:631–663.

Whitehorn, J. C. 1963. Education for uncertainty. *Perspectives in Biology and Medicine* 7:118–123.

Williams, D. D., and Garner, J. 2002. The case against "the evidence": A different perspective on evidence-based medicine. *British Journal of Psychiatry* 180:8–12.

Willick, M. S. 1993. The deficit syndrome in schizophrenia: Psychoanalytic and neurobiological perspectives. *Journal of the American Psychoanalytic Association* 41:1135–1157.

Wilson, E. O. 1998. *Consilience: The Unity of Knowledge.* New York: Vintage Books.

Yager, J. 1977. Psychiatric eclecticism: A cognitive view. *American Journal of Psychiatry* 134:736–741.

Yudofsky, S. C., and Hales, R. E. 1989. The reemergence of neuropsychiatry: Definition and direction. *Journal of Neuropsychiatry and Clinical Neurosciences* 1:3–4.

Zachar, P. 2000. Psychiatric disorders are not natural kinds. *Philosophy, Psychiatry, & Psychology* 7:167–182.

Zachar, P. 2003. The practical kinds model as a pragmatist theory of classification. *Philosophy, Psychiatry, & Psychology* 9:219–227.

Index

Printed in the United States
by Baker & Taylor Publisher Services